To _____

From _____

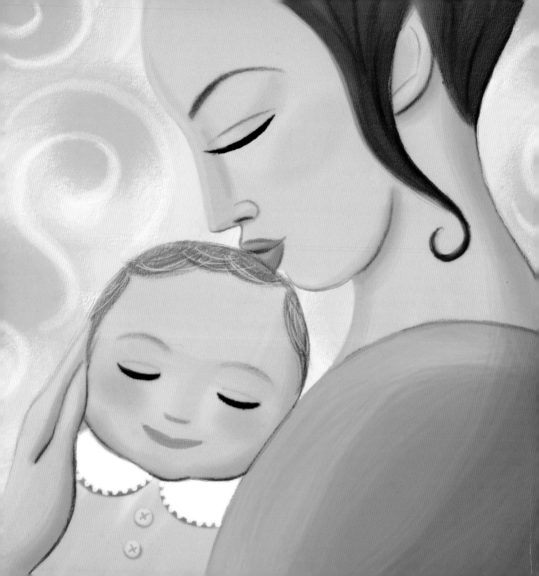

25 Things

Every Nursing Mother Needs To Know

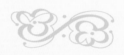

Kathleen Huggins, R.N., M.S., I.B.C.L.C.
AND Jan Ellen Brown, I.B.C.L.C.

THE HARVARD COMMON PRESS
BOSTON, MASSACHUSETTS

THE HARVARD COMMON PRESS
535 ALBANY STREET
BOSTON, MASSACHUSETTS 02118
www.harvardcommonpress.com

Printed in China
Printed on acid-free paper

Library of Congress Cataloging-in-Publication Data
Huggins, Kathleen.
25 things every nursing mother needs to know /
Kathleen Huggins and Jan Ellen Brown.
p. cm.
ISBN 978-1-55832-383-4 (hardcover)
ISBN 978-1-55832-445-9 (pbk.)
I. Breastfeeding. I. Brown, Jan Ellen, 1954- II. Title. III. Title:
Twenty-five things every nursing mother needs to know.
RJ216.H8448 2009
649'.33--dc22   2008022601

Special bulk-order discounts are available on this and other Harvard Common Press books.
Companies and organizations may purchase books for premiums or resale, or may arrange
a custom edition, by contacting the Marketing Director at the address above.

BOOK DESIGN BY DEBORAH KERNER
COVER, TITLE PAGE, AND BABY ILLUSTRATIONS BY COCO MASUDA

2   4   6   8   10   9   7   5   3   1

To our children:

Kate,

John,

KJ,

and Erin

And to our good friends and colleagues:

Ellen ("Binky") Petok

and Gretta Blythe

Contents

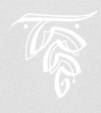

Preface

Nursing your baby can be one of your life's greatest joys. And it's best for your infant—emotionally and physically. Nursing makes the baby feel secure and nourishes her with nature's perfect food.

In the words of Dr. Grantly Dick-Read, pioneering natural-childbirth advocate and author of the groundbreaking 1944 book *Childbirth without Fear*, "The newborn baby has only three demands. They are warmth from the arms of its mother, food from her breasts, and security in the knowledge of her presence. Breastfeeding satisfies all three."

Like many women who are pregnant for the first time, you may feel anxious about breastfeeding. Your jitters may come from listening to your mother, other relatives, or friends. As you embark on the voyage of motherhood, you may feel bombarded with advice, admonitions, and rules. You may feel pressured to do everything right, including breastfeeding, but unsure what "right" means.

If you have never breastfed a baby before, it's understandable that you might question your ability to do it. Like labor and birth, breast-feeding is an unknown for you.

Relax. There are many things ahead that you can't predict or control, but you and your baby will deal with each new experience one step at a time. You will learn together.

In the meantime, you can learn about baby care and breastfeeding before the baby gets here. We have written this book to inspire you and inform you so you'll be prepared for your first weeks as a mother. The next twenty-five chapters will help you navigate the murky but buoyant waters of early motherhood. We may not be able to calm all your anxieties, but we have years of experience helping mothers and their nurslings. Let us share our insights with you.

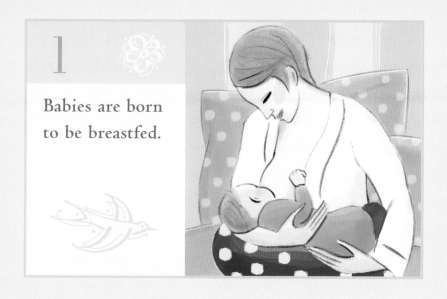

1

Babies are born
to be breastfed.

We all hear the word *bonding* associated with breast-feeding. The constant physical intimacy of breast-feeding naturally promotes the mother-baby bond, a strong and lasting psychological connection. Of course, mothers can bond with their babies regardless of how they feed their babies, but breastfeeding helps the process along. Oxytocin and prolactin, the hormones produced when you suckle your baby at your breast, flood your body with feelings of love and well-being. After the hard work of labor and birth, these hormones help both you and your baby to begin enjoying the process of nursing.

In the "quiet-alert" state that follows birth, a newborn instinctively roots for his mother's breast. When he finds it, he is rewarded with an elixir called colostrum—the special milk mothers produce for the first several days after delivery. This is your first maternal gift to your baby. The first dose of this golden milk is chock-full of antibodies, which protect the child from infection. It also carries perfect levels of sugar and protein to meet his early nutritional needs. The very act of suckling, and your milk itself, warms your baby's body and eases his transition to his new environment. Meanwhile, sucking stimulates contractions in your uterus, which in turn signal your body to start producing breast milk in earnest.

At this point, you and the baby you have dreamt about are beginning a lifelong love affair. You will marvel at his tiny fingers and toes and the way he turns toward your breast, rooting and making sucking motions with his mouth. What better way to get acquainted and to soothe him than to offer your breast? The wonder and exhilaration of childbirth melds into the joy of breastfeeding. You realize that you are now a mother, and with that revelation comes an explosion of hopes, fears, and other emotions.

The first days after your baby's birth can be a real roller-coaster ride, especially if breastfeeding doesn't come easy. Although breastfeeding is a basic maternal instinct, mothers and their babies must practice together—sometimes quite a bit—before nursing becomes second nature. Many women tell us it took weeks for them to feel comfortable nursing or to build up their milk supply. Both of us had less than perfect breastfeeding beginnings with our own babies, but in the end we were glad we waded through the doubt and fatigue. Your commitment, too, will lead to a rewarding outcome. With practice, support, and a pair of helping hands (or ears), you can breastfeed your baby!

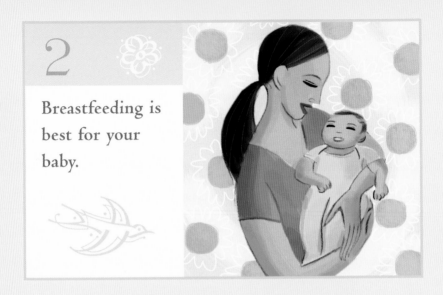

2

Breastfeeding is best for your baby.

Maybe you're still unsure whether you even *want* to breastfeed. Just as you're bound to hear scary birth stories, you'll hear your fair share of discouraging breastfeeding tales as well. You may feel pressured, afraid of being "tied down," or anxious about what your husband will think. You may worry that people will stare at you while you're nursing, that your breasts will be embarrassingly large, or that your milk will leak. If you plan on returning to work, you may be intimidated by the prospect of juggling your responsibilities. These feelings are all very common.

Health professionals tend to tiptoe around the question of breast versus formula because, they often say, they don't want a mother "to feel guilty if breastfeeding doesn't work out." It is nice if your caregiver considers your feelings, but you should know that how you feed your baby is more than just a matter of personal preference.

Is there really much of a difference between breast milk and processed infant formulas? You bet. Babies do grow on formula, of course. But scientists continually identify more and more components of breast milk that play important roles in an infant's growth and development, and formula manufacturers are continually challenged to keep up. It's unlikely that any artificial milk, whether it's based on cow's milk or soybeans, can ever duplicate nature's recipe.

Mother's milk contains proteins that promote brain development and immunities against specific human illnesses. Cow's milk, by contrast, contains proteins that favor muscle growth and immunities to bovine disease. Human babies, like all young mammals, do best with milk from their own species.

Babies on formula diets are at greater risk of illness. Diarrheal infections and respiratory illnesses are more frequent and serious among formula-fed babies. Babies deprived of breast milk tend to develop many more ear infections, which may lead to later speech and reading problems. Formula-fed infants also have higher incidences of urinary-tract infections, bacterial meningitis, colic, constipation, and allergic disorders (in fact, a significant number of babies are allergic to formulas themselves, including formulas based on soy). Babies fed only formula are more likely than breastfed babies to be hospitalized. Some studies even implicate formula feeding as one of several factors associated with sudden infant death syndrome (SIDS).

Formula feeding leads to other health problems as well. Mounting evidence indicates that artificially fed infants are at higher risk for learning disorders and generally have lower levels of intellectual functioning. Bottle-feeding with formula is associated with overfeeding and obesity, which can persist into childhood and beyond. Tooth decay, malocclusion (improper meeting of the upper and lower teeth), and distortion of the facial muscles may directly result from an infant's sucking on bottles.

Contaminants in formula pose risks, too. Formula feeding can expose a baby to toxic metals, harmful bacteria, and other toxins. High levels of aluminum have been identified in most commercial formulas. Occasionally, manufacturing errors in the production of infant formulas have resulted in product recalls.

Contamination can also occur at home, when formula is prepared for the baby. Improper storage or careless mixing can introduce harmful substances. Water used for mixing formula may be safe enough for an adult but dangerous for a baby. Some babies have suffered lead poisoning from formula diluted with tap water high in lead. Water pollution is a potential hazard even when the water is purchased in sealed bottles.

Some studies suggest that the benefits of breast over bottle extend into adulthood. On average, adults who were breastfed as infants have lower cholesterol levels, suffer less coronary artery disease, and are less prone to obesity. Other long-term benefits include protection against chronic adult digestive disorders such as Crohn's disease and ulcerative colitis. Breastfed and bottle-fed infants suffer from asthma in almost equal numbers, but adults who were breastfed as babies have a significantly lower asthma rate. Breastfeeding also decreases the chances that a baby will later develop type I diabetes or cancer of the lymph glands.

For these reasons and more, the American Academy of Pediatrics recommends that infants be offered only breast milk for the first six months after birth, and that breastfeeding continue at least through the first year. Researchers have validated what mothers (and babies) have known since the beginning of time: Breast milk is nature's formula, the perfect food for a baby, designed to meet all her nutritional needs and to protect her against illness, too. Breastfeeding is the way babies are meant to be fed.

For many reasons, of course, breastfeeding is sometimes impossible. But if you have the advantage of choosing, weigh any inhibitions you have about nursing against the proven value of breastfeeding to your baby's health and well-being. The more you consider the benefits, the less you may worry about any negatives.

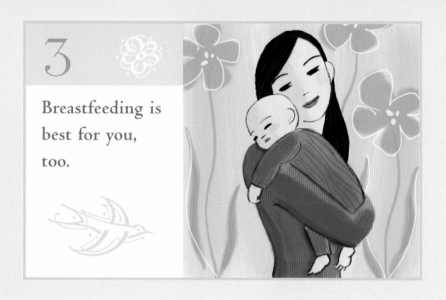

3

Breastfeeding is
best for you,
too.

Suppose we offered you something that would relax you, boost
your self-confidence, burn off calories, help you get more
rest, and provide lifelong health benefits. Oh, wait, and it is
free! Tempting, yes? Well, breastfeeding offers all this and more.

You've probably heard that breastfeeding speeds recovery after
childbirth. Nursing contracts the uterus, thus reducing the risk of

postpartum bleeding (and eventually helping to flatten your belly). And, as we mentioned in Chapter 1, breastfeeding releases hormones that relax you and promote bonding with your child. But there's more. Recent research has shown that breastfeeding provides mothers with numerous other long-term health and psychological benefits.

This should come as no surprise. After all, nursing is a natural part of the reproductive cycle. We should expect it to be the ideal mechanism for meeting the needs of infant and mother alike.

Being able to nourish your child outside the womb will give you confidence as a new mother. You'll feel secure knowing you can meet your baby's needs anytime, anywhere—and without any tools or equipment. Instead of getting up in the middle of the night to fix a bottle, you can pull your baby to your breast and doze off again. Your milk is always the right temperature, and it's always available and safe. There is no expiration date!

Any time of day, nursing provides you a reason to sit down, rest, and give your baby your undivided attention. Instead of mixing formula and washing bottles, you can relax with your child. You can leave the house without toting bottles or worrying about finding clean water. It will take a few weeks to master the art of breastfeeding, but once you do your life will be simplified.

And the benefits of breastfeeding last for the rest of your life. Studies report lower rates of ovarian cancer among women who have breastfed, and it appears that the risk of this cancer decreases the longer you nurse. Rates of premenopausal breast cancer are also lower among mothers who have breastfed. And there is mounting evidence that nursing protects women against osteoporosis (brittle bones) in later life.

Breastfeeding also delays menstruation after childbirth. Most nursing mothers go without periods for at least several months and as long as two years after delivery, provided they are nursing frequently. This makes breastfeeding a natural form of contraception.

When you nurse, you use extra calories, so you gradually lose the weight you gained during pregnancy. You shed extra pounds slowly and naturally, without any need for crash dieting. For many mothers, this is a favorite benefit of nursing.

There are financial benefits as well. You will save hundreds of dollars by not buying formula, even if you account for the cost of a breast pump and accessories.

Perhaps the most compelling reason to breastfeed is the emotional fulfillment and simple pleasure of the loving relationship that is established between mother and baby at the breast. You'll know no greater reward as a mother than witnessing your baby grow from your body—first in the womb, and then at the breast.

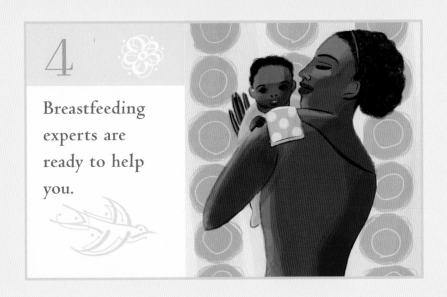

4

Breastfeeding experts are ready to help you.

Planning for your baby's arrival is exciting. You have hopes and dreams for your child and a vision of family life together. You're also preoccupied with the details and possibilities of your impending delivery. But once you've given birth, much of that anticipation is moot. You've been preparing for a major event for nine months, and suddenly it's over. So, while you're dreaming and planning, don't neglect the imminent reality of life after birth.

The first weeks with a new arrival are a time of major, though temporary, adjustment. You will need more help and advice than you did during pregnancy, and will have less time to seek it out. So give some forethought to locating breastfeeding resources that can enhance your nursing experience.

As a new mother, you are bound to get a lot of conflicting advice—some of it unsolicited—about everything to do with infant care, including breastfeeding. This can be confusing. But the old adage "The best offense is a good defense" applies here. Once you decide to breastfeed, arming yourself with credible and up-to-date information about nursing will help you sort through the chatter around you.

Knowing whom to call will streamline matters considerably when you're home with a hungry baby and have a question or concern. And having a friendly expert in your corner will give you confidence, since you'll know that help is just a phone call away.

When you interview baby doctors, discuss their philosophy about breastfeeding. Ask them what they usually recommend when a mother is having nursing difficulties. If they are truly supportive they will offer to refer you to a local lactation specialist or breastfeeding support group.

The best-known breastfeeding support group is La Leche League International (LLLI). This advocacy group was started by seven "founding mothers" in Illinois during the 1950s, when formula feeding was the norm. Through teaching and advocacy, this volunteer organization has had a profound influence on both mothers and health professionals.

Since its inception, LLLI has grown into a large and diverse organization comprising more than 7,600 volunteer leaders in sixty-five countries. Although the mission of the organization remains unchanged, La Leche now addresses an audience that is socially, economically, and culturally diverse. The LLLI website (www.llli.org) offers helpful articles in at least six languages. Many of the issues addressed in this book are discussed at the League's online forum, at http://forums.lalecheleague.org. The League's national sites, such as www.lllusa.org and www.lllc.ca, can help you locate groups and meetings in your area.

Locally, La Leche League meetings are informal discussion groups held in private homes, churches, and hospitals. There is no charge to attend a meeting, although participating parents are encouraged to become paying LLLI members. La Leche meetings are a wonderful way for pregnant women to meet new mothers and to witness women nursing babies in a relaxed setting. Local League groups usually maintain lending libraries and distribute pamphlets and other printed materials about breastfeeding.

Women who need help with their basic nursing technique or with special nursing problems can get it from a lactation specialist. Lactation specialists, or lactation consultants, are a new breed of health-care professional, trained to assess individual breastfeeding problems, provide hands-on help, and suggest special feeding strategies. Certified lactation consultants work in hospitals, doctors' offices, and WIC (Special Supplemental Nutrition Program for Women, Infants, and Children) offices. Some work in private practice. Their fees are sometimes reimbursed by medical insurers (check your plan for specific information).

Meeting with a lactation specialist is a good idea if you are experiencing any breastfeeding difficulty or if you had problems nursing a prior baby. With the specialist's help, you may find that a simple change in positioning may solve your problem. A lactation specialist can also address complicated problems that your solo efforts couldn't overcome.

An ideal way to learn about nursing is to attend a prenatal breastfeeding class. If you bring your partner, you can learn the basics together and get answers to your questions before your child is born. Besides meeting the breastfeeding expert who teaches the class, you'll learn about other local resources, and you can get referrals to baby doctors who are especially supportive of nursing moms.

Prenatal breastfeeding classes are offered by La Leche League, hospitals and birth centers, doctors, and community centers (many childbirth classes also offer a unit on breastfeeding). Usually, participants watch a video that demonstrates the way the breast makes milk and various feeding positions. Sometimes, nursing moms give demonstrations and offer their own advice.

An easy-to-read book on breastfeeding can help you learn what to expect and, after the baby is born, deal with any breastfeeding problems that may arise. Two such books stand out: *The Nursing Mother's Companion*, by Kathleen Huggins (one of the two authors of this book) and *The Womanly Art of Breastfeeding*, published by LLLI.

As with any other new skill or endeavor, breastfeeding usually comes easier if you prepare yourself well. Before long, you'll have an armful of hungry baby, and you'll be glad you planned ahead.

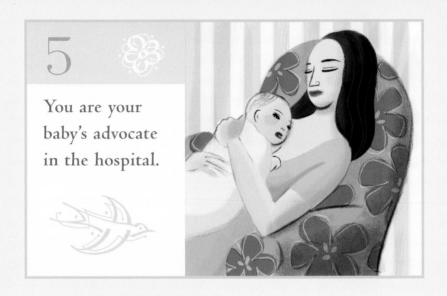

5

You are your
baby's advocate
in the hospital.

The time you spend with your baby after delivery is important, and your immediate postpartum experience can be a major factor in your breastfeeding success. If you're having your baby in a hospital or birth center, make arrangements for early nursing with the medical and support staff who attend your delivery. Well before the birth, tell your doctor or midwife and the baby's doctor that you plan to nurse your baby exclusively for the first several months. You might also discuss your intention to nurse as soon after birth as possible with the hospital or birth center's labor-and-delivery staff. If everyone involved understands your commitment to breastfeeding, they will be more likely to help you get the best start.

The birth of a baby is one of the most awesome and emotional moments of a woman's life. You will feel exhilarated afterward, but you'll also be exhausted and absorbed in the wonderment of your new baby. In all the activity of a delivery room or surgical suite, you may be tempted to put off your first nursing until everyone is done fussing around you. But experts recommend offering a baby the breast within an hour after his birth, if possible.

While you are in labor, ask the attending nurses to assist you when the time comes for the first feeding. Babies arrive well fed, but it's important to accommodate their instinct to root and attach. Put your baby to your breast as soon as he is alert and receptive. If your breast is the first thing in his mouth, he will be more inclined to nurse well later, when he enters his sleepy phase. And those first dollops of colostrum will stabilize his blood sugar, protect him from bacteria and viruses, and reduce his chance of jaundice.

You will benefit from the first nursing as well. In response to your baby's sucking, your body will release the hormone oxytocin, which will shrink your uterus and minimize your bleeding.

If, for some reason, you are unable to nurse soon after birth, don't give up. Begin nursing whenever you can, and in the meantime ask your nurse or lactation specialist to show you how to express your milk. This should be done almost immediately.

Sometimes hospital nurses will hesitate to ask a new mother to express her milk, for fear that it will "wear her out" or seem like undue pressure to start breastfeeding.

In truth, expressing your first milk doesn't take much effort. Besides, it's the second best way to get you and your baby off to a good start. The droplets of "liquid gold" colostrum can be fed to the baby via tube, spoon, or dropper, and your breasts will get the stimulation they need so they will produce plenty of milk when the baby is able to take it directly.

Mothers who are lucky enough to deliver in a Baby-Friendly hospital have a major advantage. A hospital that's been awarded the Baby-Friendly designation (by UNICEF and the World Health Organi-zation) will routinely encourage breastfeeding within an hour of birth and offer instructions for expressing milk if a baby is unable to nurse. The hospital will also discourage the use of pacifiers and avoid supplementing breast milk with formula or water unless this supplementation is medically necessary. Plus, a Baby-Friendly hospital will allow the newborn to "room in"—to stay with his mother at all times.

There may be medical reasons that you and your baby must be separated, but otherwise "rooming in" is very helpful in getting to know your baby and starting breastfeeding. Contrary to the popular notion that a new mother needs time away from her newborn to "get some rest," research has shown that mothers who room in are actually less tired than those whose babies are taken out of sight.

Your baby will be happier if you stay together, too. The baby, remember, will be experiencing an entirely new environment—one that's very different from the warm, secure, quiet, and dark surroundings of your womb. Research indicates that the best way for him to make this transition is with you—skin to skin on your chest or very close by, where he can sense your presence.

The practice of holding a baby skin to skin, sometimes known as "kangaroo care," is as simple and easy as it sounds. It is also extremely beneficial to your newborn. Placed against your chest, your baby will be warmed by your body and will be able to smell and hear you. (Dad can hold the baby this way, too.)

Mothers of premature babies are commonly told to hold their babies skin to skin even if wires and tubes are attached to the newborn, because preemies who have had this intimate experience have been shown to better maintain their body temperature, heart rate, and respiratory rate, and to grow faster. They also have an easier time learning to breastfeed, when they are ready.

When you need help with breastfeeding, ask for it. Get up in a chair, and practice positioning with an experienced nurse or lactation specialist. Have her teach you how to lie on your side to nurse. If your baby is sleepy or you are having any nipple or breast pain, let your helper know. The squeaky wheel gets the oil, in the hospital as elsewhere. It's better to insist on having someone monitor multiple feeding attempts than to go home unprepared. Be prepared to work a bit to get the advice and instruction you need.

You can expect many interruptions during your time in the hospital. Many hospitals have relaxed their visiting hours, so well-meaning visitors are more likely to drop in. A recent study reviewed the number of interruptions during the hospital stay of twenty-nine brand-new moms who intended to breastfeed. The researchers kept track of the number and duration of visits and phone calls, both medical and personal, between 8 A.M. and 8 P.M. On average, the new mothers experienced fifty-four visits or phone calls *per day*. Only one-fourth of the interruptions were by the nursing staff. Nurses, of course, need to interrupt sometimes; visitors are another matter. When you should be recovering and learning the art of breastfeeding, you don't need to play hostess. Have your partner or another family member or friend act as a gatekeeper, discouraging casual visitors or at least limiting their stays. Ask your nurses to minimize interruptions during naps and nursing times (but do take all the breastfeeding help you can get).

A mother's primary responsibility is to ensure the best for her children. You will be your baby's advocate throughout his life. By starting now, you will ensure his well-being and comfort and provide him with the best start in life. Don't hesitate to play an active role in his amazing first days.

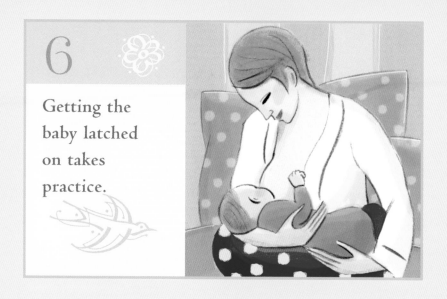

6

Getting the
baby latched
on takes
practice.

There is a good reason that lactation specialists make so much ado about "latch-on." If your baby sucks at your breast without latching on properly, he won't get as much milk as he should, and you'll suffer increasing discomfort. He may get frustrated and pull off the nipple repeatedly, or he may gradually slide off the breast until his tongue creases the nipple. Once your nipple is hurting and you're anticipating more pain, you may be too hesitant to get the baby latched on well. Soon you may wonder which came first: the pain from a poor latch or a poor latch because you are in pain.

Did you learn to ride a bike the first time you got on one? Or whistle or tie your shoes on the first attempt? Positioning the baby for feedings and getting him latched on to the breast are like any new skills; it will take time for you and your baby to master them. With practice and perseverance, latching your baby to your breast can become second nature to both of you.

The only way to really learn this skill is with your baby at your breast. It helps, however, to study the basics before you give birth. In a prenatal breastfeeding class, your instructor will explain the principles and describe various positions. If you attend a La Leche League meeting, babies and mothers who have mastered the skill of latching will demonstrate it. It will look so easy that you'll wonder why there is so much fuss about it.

Just knowing that this skill takes time and patience to master can make the learning period easier for you and your baby. Some mothers and babies enjoy a perfect fit from the start. This shouldn't surprise you; after all, babies were born to nurse. Breastfeeding is indeed one of our most basic natural functions. For any number of reasons, however, latching on to the breast doesn't always come so naturally.

Very soon after birth, your baby will instinctively root and scramble for the breast. Nipples come in all shapes and sizes, but your baby has no idea there are different models. He will look for your areola (the dark ring of skin around your nipple), and it will become his reference for future nursing.

Your nurse can help you direct your baby to your nipple. Wait patiently until the baby opens his mouth wide—don't worry, he will—and then draw him to your breast. If you don't score on the first attempt, adjust your position. Try any position that keeps his tummy against yours, so that he doesn't have to twist his neck or body to nurse. Align his nose with your nipple, with his jaw away from the nipple itself. Then, when you pull him onto the breast, your nipple will land in the baby's palate and trigger his sucking.

Previous generations of women were taught to cradle a baby in the crook of an arm and offer a nipple by clamping it between two fingers, scissors-like. This technique did not provide the best latch, and women's nipples would become sore as a result. When that happened, they were told that their nipples needed "toughening" or that the babies were nursing too long. (The latter may have been true, since an improper latch can slow the flow of milk.) Fortunately for all concerned, babies often corrected their latch themselves, and the nursings improved. Many women, though, gave up and turned to the bottle.

If you start out nursing with your baby latched on right, not only will you avoid nipple soreness and injury, but you will set a pattern for future nursing and start building your milk supply.

How do you judge whether your baby is latched on well? The main criteria are comfort and efficacy. If your baby is sucking well and you are not in pain, then you most likely have an effective latch. You may feel some tenderness and maybe even some pinching at the beginning of a feeding session, but otherwise nursing shouldn't hurt.

When the baby's sucking slows, break the suction, if necessary, by placing a finger inside the corner of the baby's mouth and gently pressing down. Although not every baby burps after nursing, give him the opportunity by placing him over your shoulder or by holding him sitting up with your hand supporting his chin and back. Once he has burped, change his diaper, if needed, and then offer your other breast.

Continue nursing until the baby is no longer actively sucking. Don't keep track of the amount of time spent at each breast. Feedings usually range from twenty to forty-five minutes in length, but they may be shorter or longer.

After the feeding, check the condition of your nipples. They will likely be a bit elongated. That's natural. But creased, wedged, smushed, and beveled nipples are all signs that the nipple wasn't far enough back in the baby's mouth. A shallow latch can lead to soreness for Mom and low milk intake for the baby.

If your baby can't latch on well—perhaps because of the way his mouth or your nipple is formed—a visit with a lactation specialist will be invaluable. She can evaluate your situation and teach you techniques to improve your baby's latch. She can also advise you how to protect your milk supply until your baby can latch on better.

If your nipples become cracked or abraded, seek treatment right away. You will need advice on healing remedies and, most important, you'll need to learn to correct the latch. Nipple injury can lead to breast engorgement and infection (mastitis), which can result in an unnecessary weaning.

If your nipples are so injured that you can't nurse your baby, express your milk and feed it by bottle or dropper until you can resume breastfeeding comfortably. Milk removal is the key to milk production, and pumping or hand expression will maintain your supply until you are healed.

How can you be sure that the baby is getting milk? For the first few days after birth, your breasts will produce only small quantities of colostrum, and your baby won't swallow as much as he will when your mature milk comes in. But soon you'll be able to hear or see your baby swallow. Listen to the sounds he makes as he nurses. Just after latching on, he'll take several short, choppy sucks; this is when your toes curl if you have sore nipples. Then he'll launch into long, slow sucks. Some babies are not very audible swallowers—we call them stealth nursers—but if you can't hear swallowing you should at least be able to see the long drawing motion of the baby's jaw (wiggling ears indicate sucking, not swallowing). This jaw motion shows you that the baby is taking in milk.

You may be confused if someone asks you if your milk is "letting down." How can you know? Oxytocin, the hormone that triggered the production of colostrum soon after the birth, is released every time your baby begins to nurse. Once you're producing milk, this hormone triggers what's called the let-down reflex. It causes the milk stored in your breasts to flow through your milk ducts to the pores (yes, you have more than one) in your nipples. Women often feel their milk let down, but most don't feel the sensation strongly when they first start breastfeeding. Rest assured, if your baby is sucking well and gaining weight, your milk is letting down.

As experienced mothers will tell you, every baby has her own nursing style. You may have a sleepy baby, a grazer, a gourmet, or a barracuda. Regardless, in a short time the two of you will develop a rhythm and style that works for both of you.

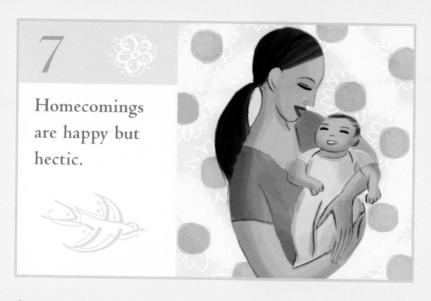

7

Homecomings are happy but hectic.

The first days at home after childbirth are a time for recuperation and adjustment. You need quiet to attend to your newborn's needs as well as to your own. Planning ahead can help make your first weeks at home a memory you will cherish forever. Your goal is to create a calm and supportive environment in which you, your family, and your new baby can get to know each other.

Before labor begins, start preparing a nursing nook—a comfortable and secure spot for nursing. Your nook can be a rocker, glider, couch, or bed with a small table beside it. Arrange your nook so you'll have anything you're likely to need within arm's reach—water or juice, nutritious snacks, a phone and a list of important numbers, the TV remote or books or magazines, paper and pencils, a nursing pillow, and, if you need to use one, a breast pump. If you plan to do most of your nursing in a room far from the kitchen, you might even invest in a dorm-size refrigerator to minimize interruptions and trips back and forth for supplies.

If you're leaving the hospital within forty-eight hours after the birth, your milk may not be "in" yet—that is, your breasts may still be producing colostrum, not mature milk. In this case, make an appointment to see the baby's doctor or a lactation specialist in a day or two. Plan to nurse the baby often, keep a record of feedings and of wet and soiled diapers, and jot down questions to ask the doctor.

Caring for a new baby is time consuming and physically taxing.

You simply won't be able to fall back into familiar household routines. Coming home to a sink full of dirty dishes, unmade beds, and a pile of dirty laundry would distract you from settling in and nursing your baby. You'll feel better if you feel in control, and you'll feel more in control if your home isn't a mess. But your priority is your baby. You'll therefore need the help of your partner, family, and possibly an outside cleaning service to keep the areas of your home you use the most clean and uncluttered.

Delegating household tasks to friends and relatives is one way to make sure you'll be able to relax—*if* your helpers don't move in with you. Many couples have house guests waiting for them when they bring their babies home. These extra pairs of hands are meant to manage the household, provide experienced baby care, and run errands. But the helpers can also get in the way. If you have enough space, have live-in visitors sleep in a private room, to which they can retreat at times to give everyone some privacy. If space is tight, consider accommodating your helpers in a nearby hotel. In either case, make your expectations for your guests clear. You want to avoid conflict and tension at a time when shifting hormones, physical discomfort, and fatigue can combine to frazzle your nerves.

Although you may be delighted to be back in your own home, the postbirth adrenaline that got you to this point is wearing off, and you may find yourself on that famous emotional roller coaster. The biggest event of your life has just taken place, and you are beginning to realize the magnitude of being a mother. You may miss the support of hospital staff.

Your first night home can be especially difficult. Just knowing this may help you get through.

Be assured that things will change—in ways that may surprise you. That tiny baby who was so sleepy in the hospital may suddenly become lively. We could retire if we had a dollar for every time a new mother has told us, "She has her days and nights mixed up. She sleeps all days and fusses and nurses all night!"

Or maybe your baby is sleeping so much that both day and night feedings are infrequent. In this case, offer your breast whenever the baby stirs or her eyelids flutter. Undress her, and hold her against your bare skin. If she seems lethargic or difficult to rouse, or isn't regularly wetting and soiling diapers, call the baby's doctor. Don't worry about being labeled a nervous new mother; it is better to be told that the baby is fine than to risk letting a small problem turn into a bigger one.

Somewhere between day two and day four after birth, you will probably notice that your breasts are full or even downright swollen. When this happens, you should nurse more often to keep the engorgement from worsening.

If the usually pliable areola tissue and nipple are stretched tight from engorgement, you may have trouble getting or keeping the baby latched on to your breast. She may bob and weave as she tries to find something she can grasp. What a frustrating time! Your milk supply is increasing, but the baby is having trouble nursing. Try pressing with your fingers on the area around the base of your nipple to push the swelling back, away from your nipple, so your baby can take more of the areola into her mouth. Or relieve the pressure by expressing some of your milk.

When you get the baby latched on, stroke and massage your breasts while she sucks to help your milk flow. If your baby quickly falls asleep while nursing or sucks weakly, compress your breasts to help empty them: Place your thumb across the top of your breast, cradle the underside with your fingers, and squeeze gently when your baby pauses to swallow.

If despite your efforts to relieve the engorgement your baby still cannot latch on, pump or hand-express some milk into a spoon, and carefully put the tip of the spoon to your baby's lips. She may be able to take some milk that way. If this doesn't work, offer her your milk from a dropper or bottle.

If your engorgement is severe, cold compresses may ease your discomfort. Some women use cold green cabbage leaves to suppress inflammation (yes, vegetables in the bra!).

Remember, mild engorgement is normal; it means the production of mature milk has begun on schedule. If your breasts do not feel fuller by the fourth day after childbirth, consult a lactation specialist, and have your baby's weight checked.

Your first days at home with your new baby may be rocky as well as exhilarating. Although there is no sure-fire recipe for postpartum bliss, getting your house in order and putting your support system in place before the birth will go a long way in helping you navigate the early days of motherhood.

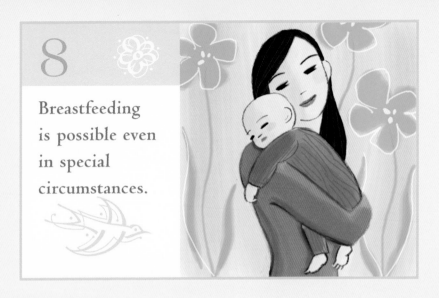

8

Breastfeeding
is possible even
in special
circumstances.

In the course of our work as lactation counselors, we routinely help mothers facing complications resulting from multiple or premature births. We deal with adoptive families and babies born to surrogate mothers, as well as newborns facing a variety of medical risks and special needs. We know this: Whatever your situation, your desire to hold your baby (or babies) to your breast can usually be met.

You will have to learn and accept special guidelines to match your situation, but understanding breastfeeding basics is a good place to start. If you learn during pregnancy that you'll face special challenges, you should attend regular prenatal breastfeeding classes. You may at times feel frustrated because you know that the information presented won't necessarily apply to you and your baby, but you'll be building a solid foundation for you own nursing experience. Understanding the fundamentals of latching, positioning, and milk production will prepare you for whatever's to come. These classes can also put you in touch with the special local resources you will need.

Since we began our careers, the most profound advances made in treating newborns have been in the area of prematurity. Today preemies are much likelier to survive and develop well. Research, technology, and experience have given babies born too early a better start than at any other time in history.

Many studies have shown that breast milk and the act of breast-feeding are among the best therapies for preemies. In fact, nursing can be vital to a preemie's short- and long-term health. On a diet of mother's milk, premature babies are better protected from respiratory and digestive infections and grow faster.

The days after giving birth to a premature baby can be overwhelming, particularly if your baby is sick or very immature. You may have doubts about many things, including your ability to nurse your baby. If your baby can't take your milk directly from your breast, a lactation specialist or experienced nurse or doctor can show you how to pump your breasts and collect and store your milk, which can be fed to the baby by bottle or other means.

If your premature baby has ups and downs, you may feel very discouraged at times. But you may also find satisfaction in being able to provide what your baby needs most—your milk—when he is most vulnerable.

You'll feel the same satisfaction if you breastfeed an adopted baby or one who was carried by a surrogate. Yes, even women who have never been pregnant can breastfeed. Many do this with the aid of a device that delivers formula or donor milk to the baby through a feeding tube taped to the mother's breast. Some women actually induce lactation, through hand expression or pumping and, sometimes, herbs or prescription drugs that stimulate milk production. If you want to try this, find a health professional who has experience in inducing lactation. She can explain your options and refer you to adoptive mothers who can share their experiences with you.

What if your milk has "dried up"? This happens sometimes in the early weeks. Perhaps you had trouble nursing and had poor advice. Or perhaps you decided to stop nursing, only to find that your baby was allergic to formula. Or perhaps you just changed your mind about how you wanted to feed your baby. In any case, stimulating your breasts and expressing new milk can restart milk production (this is called "relactation").

Extra breast stimulation can also help women who have undergone cosmetic or reconstructive breast surgery or suffered injury or trauma to the endocrine system. Such women—and especially those who have had breast reductions—often struggle to provide a full milk supply for their babies. Diana West, who nursed three sons after breast-reduction surgery, hosts a website called BFAR.org, for Breast Feeding After Reduction. West maintains that there are "many means of maximizing the milk-producing capability of any portion of the mammary system that remains intact and functional." Breastfeeding is possible after a breast reduction, West concludes, if you have at least one breast with a nipple and areola.

And what if you're expecting twins or triplets? Mothers of multiples are sometimes restricted to bed rest during pregnancy. They also frequently have surgical or premature deliveries, or both. These complications, combined with the obvious challenges of mothering two, three, or more babies, can tempt a mother to give up on breastfeeding. But didn't nature give us two breasts so we can nurse two babies at once?

Seriously, there are many resources available to help you. Talk with other mothers who have nursed multiple newborns. Look for the many books, videos, classes, and websites devoted to the subject of breastfeeding after a multiple birth. There are even national and local Mothers of Multiples groups. If you know you're pregnant with multiples, you can take advantage of these resources even before you give birth.

The baby with a birth defect may need his mother's milk and the comfort and security of her breast even more than other infants. The birth of a baby with a cardiac defect, a cleft lip or palate, or any other genetic or developmental condition is understandably a time of confusion and shock for the family. But by holding the baby skin to skin at your breast and providing your life-sustaining milk, you will both comfort him and help yourself to accept his condition and move forward in your mothering journey.

If you are dealing with any of these challenges, we strongly recommend getting support from a lactation specialist. However overwhelming your circumstances as a new mother, with good help you may still be able to breastfeed.

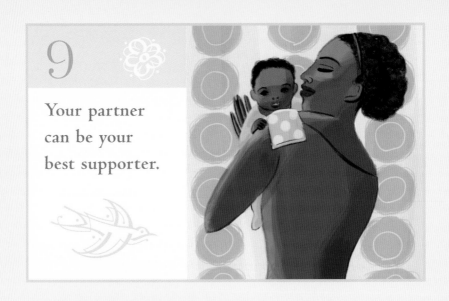

9

Your partner
can be your
best supporter.

Perhaps the most important piece of advice we can offer new
mothers is this: include your partner in every aspect of child
care—from pregnancy to birth and through college.

"Your partner" can be anyone who is on hand when the baby
arrives and available to help you in the weeks and years that follow.

(Although we refer to your partner as *he*, yours may of course be female.)

Because breastfeeding promotes a special bond between mother and baby, your partner may feel left out. In a way, he *is* left out. Breastfeeding mothers and babies enter their own orbit; their symbiotic relationship seems almost magical to others.

Although your baby is your first concern, your partner will be more supportive if you help him to feel he is part of the team. And he does have a role to play in nurturing your baby. Like you, he is falling in love with the baby. And he is the key to maintaining a harmonious household during your baby's first weeks at home.

The more your partner knows about baby care, the more help he will be—in practical ways such as changing diapers and in less tangible ways such as giving you encouragement. Robert and James Sears's companion book in this series, *Father's First Steps: 25 Things Every New Dad Should Know*, makes a good gift for a partner. It discusses every aspect of caring for a baby, with emphasis on support for breastfeeding. Some hospitals and birth centers offer classes just for new dads, on all aspects of early fatherhood. You might look for such a class in your community.

When women have difficulties breastfeeding, some partners quickly suggest switching to the bottle. Your partner won't do this if he has been schooled in the benefits of nursing and has learned tactics to overcome rough spots. Twenty years ago, fathers came to our breastfeeding classes begrudgingly and averted their eyes when we showed videos or demonstrated breast pumps. But in the past decade we've noticed partners taking more active roles in these classes and sometimes asking the best questions. If you take a breastfeeding class, be sure your partner is on hand to learn the hows and whys of nursing with you.

In the delivery room, your partner can play an important role by reminding the staff about your intention to breastfeed and by preventing unnecessary interruptions. He can graciously but firmly deflect visitors and delay nonurgent hospital procedures while both of you spend time getting acquainted with the baby.

The sooner your partner holds the baby (and he too can take off his shirt to hold the baby against his skin), the less awkward he will feel in his new role. A newborn can seem vulnerable and fragile. The sooner your partner learns he will not crush or drop the squirming bundle, the better off you all will be.

Once your partner witnesses the baby rooting for your breast, he'll truly comprehend the magnitude of the breastfeeding relationship. He can help with feedings by unwrapping the baby and gently waking her by massaging her or slowly lifting her into a sitting position. He can place pillows to support you. He can place the baby with her tummy against yours and her nose to your nipple so she will be in place to latch on. He can hold her little fists so they don't compete with your nipple. This may all seem silly to you if you are still pregnant, but, take our word for it, you will be grateful your partner is there in the first days of nursing.

However bleary-eyed he may be, your partner should be present at early feedings supervised by a nurse or lactation specialist. This way he can mentally file away tricks of the trade to remind you of later.

Your partner can be a great soother and burper. He can be the first person to show your baby that love does not always involve food. And he'll love doing this. We have seen many a dad beam from ear to ear when he picks up a fussy baby and soothes and quiets her.

Probably the most common question partners ask in class is, "When can I feed the baby a bottle?" This is not a ploy to undermine nursing or to take the baby away from the mother. It usually is just what it sounds like: A question of when Dad can feed the baby, too. Our response goes something like this: "Once the baby is nursing well and has little trouble latching on to the breast, an occasional bottle usually does no harm." (If you skip a nursing, though, it is essential to express your milk instead.)

If you will be returning to work soon, you will need to introduce a bottle and get the baby used to being fed by someone besides yourself. Your partner can be very helpful in the process. The baby may be more willing to take the bottle from him than from you. And your partner can show other people how to hold the baby in an upright position for feeding, so she takes milk slowly instead of guzzling.

Never forget that your partner needs time with the baby, and that you need him to have this time. His support is important to you, and if you don't anticipate it, foster it, and embrace it, you may unwittingly discourage it. You're the one with the breastfeeding bond, but your partner needs to develop his own special relationship with the baby as well.

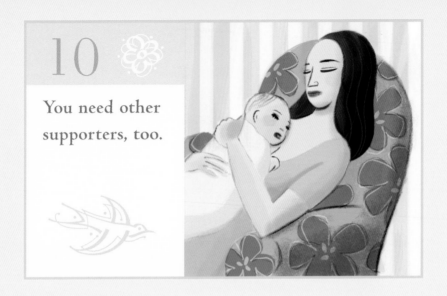

10

You need other supporters, too.

Although most American women know that breastfeeding is best for their babies, more than half who begin nursing give up and switch to bottle-feeding within a few months. There are many reasons for this, but too many women give up simply because they lack a support network. It's normal for mothers to question the decision to breastfeed, especially during the first few weeks, but things improve after that. (Honest!) So we encourage you to surround yourself with people who understand and respect the breastfeeding relationship, who support your intentions, and who will cater to your needs until breastfeeding is easy for you.

Your partner, family, and friends all play roles in supporting you as a nursing mother. On days when you're exhausted, frustrated, or discouraged, friends and family members can serve as good listeners and help you get back on track. If they have read up on breastfeeding or attended prenatal classes, they'll understand the importance of being patient and persistent during the first weeks after delivery.

Friends who have breastfed their own babies can be both a blessing and a curse. Most mothers can remember the fatigue and discouragement of their own early days and can give you the pep talks you need. But a "dairy queen" who pumped pints of milk at a time may not commiserate with your fledgling milk supply. Worse may be a friend whose advice reflects her own struggle but has nothing to do with your own. Beware especially of friends for whom breastfeeding did not work out. They may offer a shoulder to cry on when times are tough, but they may unconsciously undermine your progress as they wrestle with the loss of their own breastfeeding relationship. An offhand comment like "I gave my babies formula, and they turned out all right" can send you over the edge if you are feeling emotional, fatigued, or discouraged. Keep a sense of humor, and remember that people love to give advice, even when they may not know much about a subject.

From older people especially, be prepared for unsolicited advice like "You're going to spoil him by holding him all the time" and "He's just using you as a pacifier; he must not be getting enough milk." Nonsense! These ideas were born when women gave birth sedated and were routinely separated from their babies, who were given pacifiers and bottles on strict four-hour schedules. As a new mother, you will probably find such advice counterintuitive, but it may have such a familiar ring that it may cause you to doubt yourself and your baby. Remember, you are the one who observes your baby's every expression and movement. He is telling you, not your grand-mother, what he needs. As long as you're comfortable and your baby is growing, you can trust your body and your child. You are the fore-most expert on your baby.

Your family members are as concerned about you as they are about the baby. If they see you and the baby struggling, they'll naturally want to "fix" the problem and restore equilibrium to the household. If they have concerns or fears about nursing, address their miscon-ceptions with the information you gained in prenatal or breastfeed-ing classes. Discussing their concerns calmly and logically will help defuse any mounting tension.

If your family sees you struggling with more than the common "baby blues" for a few weeks after birth, their concern may be well placed. Some women experience serious emotional problems after childbirth. If you are in the midst of a postpartum depressive or anx-iety episode, you may be the last to recognize the symptoms.

If you experience a change in appetite and sleep patterns, obsessive worry or guilt feelings and concern for the baby, a lack of energy, panic attacks, or frequent episodes of crying, let your family and friends lead you to a professional who can evaluate and treat you. If medication is suggested, ask for one that is compatible with breast-feeding (and many are). In the past, anxious mothers were encouraged to wean. But new research suggests that salvaging the breastfeeding relationship is therapeutic for mother and baby during an episode of anxiety or depression.

Every new mother sometimes questions her mothering abilities and decisions. Informed and supportive people around you can encourage you, and they can help you learn to trust your mothering instincts and intuition. Let your partner and all your loved ones know how much their support means to you. With a little help from your friends, you will survive, and your baby will thrive.

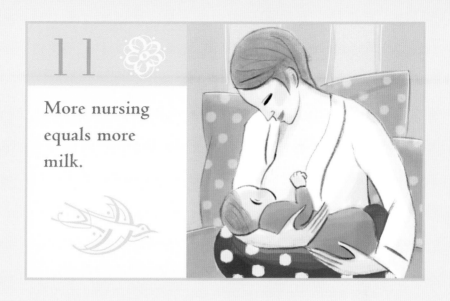

11

More nursing equals more milk.

We are mammals—members of the class of animals defined by our ability to provide milk to our young. So you might think that any new mother would pour forth an ample supply of breast milk effortlessly. Unfortunately, it doesn't work that way. The flow of milk must be prompted and then sustained.

The prompting comes from your baby the first time he latches on to your breast. Increasing and then sustaining the flow requires that you empty your breasts frequently and thoroughly. Initiating a steady flow of milk early in your breastfeeding career will guarantee your having the optimum supply until you stop nursing, no matter how your baby's needs change.

During the last months of pregnancy, your body produces and stores that miracle food, colostrum. When your baby nurses for the first time, he receives his first inoculation of sorts. Along with the immunities passed to him via the placenta, he receives insurance doses in your colostrum, and later your mature milk, to carry him through until his own immune system can take over months later.

Something else very important happens during that initial nursing. The baby's sucking stimulates nerves that send a message to your endocrine system. They say it's time to produce more colostrum and, very soon, mature milk.

The system works by supply and demand. Your baby (or an effective pump) demands a supply by stimulating the nipple and, in turn, the pituitary gland. This sets in motion the process of ongoing milk production.

Sounds simple, right? It is, if you remember the underlying principle of milk production: Remove it or lose it. This means nursing soon after birth, if only momentarily, even if labor and delivery were rough. It means keeping the baby in the room with you and not down the hall in the nursery. It means you can't skip breast-milk feedings because Dad, Grandma, or anyone else wants to feed the baby. Do we sound pushy? Well, we've seen too many mothers get off to a poor start when early feedings and milk removal could have ensured future supply. As La Leche League says, "early and often" is the rule in nursing newborns.

There's a sound physiological reason for this. Research shows that breast milk contains a substance called the *feedback inhibitor of lactation* (FIL). This peptide does exactly what its clumsy name implies. When you leave milk in your breasts, FIL causes your milk-producing cells to shrink, and this slows production. This is how women "dry up" their milk deliberately: You just leave milk in the breast, and it eventually disappears—and you stop making more. This can also happen unintentionally, if you neglect to empty your breasts often, especially in the early days after delivery. When women complain of a low milk supply after several weeks of nursing, we can often trace the problem back to a few early days of sketchy nursing or pumping.

So, nurse frequently, at least eight times per day. You don't have to space the feeding evenly over the day and night; many babies prefer to bunch several feedings close together and then sleep for long intervals. During feedings, watch for active swallowing, and check that your breasts are softer or lighter afterward; these are both signs that your baby is consuming milk. Switch breasts during a feeding when the first one softens; this will ensure that at least one breast is emptied at each feeding, and also that your baby will get a good mixture of high-sugar foremilk and fatty, satiating hindmilk.

People may tell you to never wake a sleeping baby, and that she will wake up if she is hungry. Usually she will. But, in the early days, when you are "phoning in your order" for milk, following such advice can upset the milk cart. Some newborns will sleep right through feedings if you let them. If your baby is nursing less than eight times per day, wake her for feedings every three hours.

You may become concerned about your milk supply if your baby seems hungry after feedings or nurses for long periods and never seems satisfied. If your baby is frequently wetting and soiling diapers, she is likely getting enough milk. Her bowel movements should be bigger than a spoonful, and they should change from black to brown or greenish by the fourth day after birth, and to yellow by the fifth day. Your baby's urine may be scant during the first few days, but it should be more frequent and clear by day five.

A doctor or lactation professional can confirm that your baby is getting enough milk by weighing her. Newborns normally lose a little weight during the first few days after birth, but by the fifth day they should begin gaining about an ounce a day. Most babies regain their birth weight by day fourteen.

Don't make the mistake of comparing your milk output to the amount your baby will take from a bottle. You may pump three to four ounces from your breasts at a time, but see her drink four to five ounces from a bottle. Babies often take more from bottles, because milk flows faster from a bottle. Just as adults sometimes continue to eat after they're no longer hungry, your baby may take more than she actually needs when the milk is readily available.

If you find out that your milk supply is inadequate, this is probably because your baby isn't emptying your breasts at each feeding. There are many possible causes of this problem. The baby may not be able to latch on well because she is tongue-tied or has a high palate, or because your nipples are inverted or flattened. Babies born before thirty-eight weeks gestation often lack the stamina or energy to complete a feeding. The same is true of sleepy and jaundiced babies. Such problems call for a visit with a lactation specialist, who can assess the problem and help in developing a feeding plan.

Sometimes the cause of a low milk supply is less obvious. There are red flags we look for: no significant change in breast size during pregnancy; a history of infertility associated with endocrine problems, insulin resistance, or thyroid disorder; a history of a low milk supply with another baby; and previous breast injury, breast surgery, or chest trauma.

We have seen mothers with a wide variety of breast sizes and shapes who have no milk-production problems whatsoever. Some flat-chested mothers feed twins and triplets. But although breast size doesn't affect the ability to produce milk, women with larger breasts may be able to *store* more milk. Large-breasted women may enjoy longer intervals between feedings because they deliver more milk at each. Small-breasted mothers may deliver smaller quantities of milk at each feeding and so may need to nurse more often to meet their babies' needs.

Recently lactation specialists have linked low milk supply to the resurgence of scheduled feedings. Popular books about "parent-directed breastfeeding" promise, seductively, that you can "get them to sleep through the night." But expecting a baby to nurse according to a schedule usually leads to frustration for both mother and baby—and sometimes to breastfeeding failure.

Once your milk supply is established and you're nursing your baby whenever she seems hungry, a natural rhythm will probably emerge. Until then, if you cut back on nursing sessions or skip feedings to suit yourself, you may drastically reduce your milk production.

After nursing is established, your baby will have growth spurts and associated appetite spurts. At these times your baby will nurse more often, and this in turn will cause you to produce more milk. Your supply will soon meet the increased demand.

So, go with the flow. Remember that more nursing equals more milk, and seek help if your milk supply seems low.

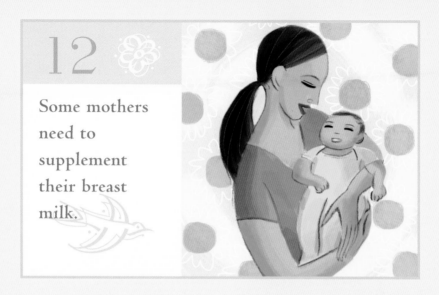

12

Some mothers need to supplement their breast milk.

Although most women who find they don't have enough milk can be helped with a few adjustments in the way they nurse, as outlined in Chapter 11, some mothers may need to beef up their babies' diet with formula or, better, donated mother's milk.

Available from milk banks throughout North America (your lactation specialist can refer you to the nearest), donor milk is the preferred dietary supplement for babies. Unfortunately, the milk is expensive and, unless the baby is sick, usually not covered by health insurance. If donor milk is not an option for you, ask your baby's doctor to recommend an appropriate formula.

Your pediatrician or family doctor will monitor your baby's weight and growth. Babies who are exclusively breastfed should gain four to seven ounces per week for the first several months. Older babies should gain two to three ounces per week. After the first months, a doctor tracks a baby's length and the circumference of his head as well as his weight. If your breastfed baby is not growing as expected, the doctor should refer you to a lactation specialist.

During a typical visit, a lactation specialist will review the baby's birth and feeding history, examine your breasts and the baby's mouth and jaw, and observe a feeding (these appointments are ideally scheduled for when a baby is likely to be hungry).

There are two factors at play here: the amount of milk you produce and the amount of milk your baby consumes at a feeding.

During the past decade, lactation specialists have developed a fairly reliable method for taking both into account.

Using very precise scales, lactation specialists weigh the baby before and after a feeding. The difference in the baby's two weights tells them how much milk the baby took during the feeding. Then they pump the mother's breasts and measure how much milk was left at the end of the feeding. The sum of these two measurements roughly equals the mother's total milk supply. The results will depend partially on the time of day, the baby's disposition, the length of the feeding, and, especially, how much time has passed since the preceding feeding. But the method provides approximate figures that allow a comparison between the mother's milk supply and the baby's ability to remove the available milk.

Don't try this method with your bathroom or kitchen scale; it isn't precise enough. If your baby is premature or clearly has feeding problems, you can rent a scale so you can track his intake at home.

Many breastfeeding advocates feel that this comparative-weight method is "too scientific" and fear that it could undermine a nursing mother's confidence. But studies show that the method actually relieves women's anxiety and helps them to resolve feeding problems.

If your lactation specialist determines that you're producing enough milk but your baby isn't taking it all from your breasts, you can continue nursing as before, but you can also pump your breasts for about ten minutes after each nursing and offer the baby your residual milk by bottle.

If the baby needs more milk than you are producing, you can do the same thing, but add donor milk or formula to the bottle. Be sure to nurse until the baby's swallowing slows. While you nurse, compress your breasts to maximize the flow of milk. Afterward, offer the bottle slowly, so the baby swallows only a little at a time.

If you don't have time for both nursing and pumping, you can pump all your milk and offer it to your baby by bottle, with or without a supplement, as needed. This may be necessary if for some reason your baby can't latch on or suck effectively.

Christina Smillie, a noted pediatrician, recommends giving a baby a supplemental bottle just *before* offering him the breast. This satiates his thirst and gives him a full feeling, and he comes to associate these sensations with latching on and suckling. Women who have tried this method like it because feedings conclude at the breast. The mother and baby can cuddle as long as they like, and the baby can drift off to sleep.

If you prefer to avoid bottles entirely or use them as little as possible, you can breastfeed and supplement your baby's diet simultaneously by using a device specially designed for this purpose. It consists of a plastic bag or rigid container that you fill with milk or formula and wear around your neck, and a thin tube that runs from the bag to your nipple. The baby can take both the tube and your nipple into his mouth and so stimulate your breast while taking milk from the tube. Some women find these "supplementers" clumsy, unnatural, and ultimately too frustrating to use, but other women say the devices are the answer to their prayers.

Sometimes the reasons for a mother's low milk supply are obvious; other times they're a muddled combination of factors—a poor start, a sleepy baby who doesn't let Mom know he's hungry, a busy mother who misses cues. Sometimes illness, the mother's or the baby's, disrupts the process of building a milk supply. Nursing may have started out well but gotten derailed.

Whatever the reason your baby isn't getting enough milk, don't blame yourself. Supplementing your milk is not a sign you have failed as a mother. Focus on the goal of getting sufficient food into your baby, however you have to do it. Once your baby gets back on track, he'll have more energy to nurse. His appetite will be more predictable, and you can stop worrying about how much milk he is getting.

Even if you have to feed a lot of supplement, you can continue to nurse as long as the baby is willing and able. And he will benefit from every drop of your milk that he gets.

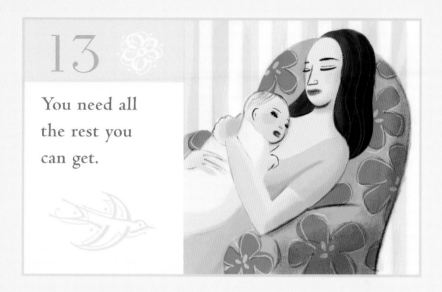

13

You need all the rest you can get.

At some point in your breastfeeding career, you'll probably say that your baby won't let you get enough sleep. After worries about getting the baby latched on to the breast and milk supply, sleep deprivation is the most common concern of new mothers.

While you were pregnant, you may have been frequently awakened by kicking, squirming, and things that go bump in the womb. You likely had to get up to make repeated trips to the bathroom as your baby competed for space with your bladder. You may have tossed and turned in bed to find a comfortable position to sleep in. We call all this a dress rehearsal for motherhood. Breastfeeding mothers are on call around the clock.

A baby's sleep-wake cycle may vary throughout the course of the day, but it never stops. And when a baby wakes up, she wants to be fed. Further, many babies like to escape bustle and noise during the day by sleeping and then rock and roll all night, causing their mothers to conclude their infants have day and night mixed up. This can be tough on Mom.

As their children grow up, many mothers hold fond memories of nighttime nursings. The warmth, the intimacy, the baby's breath against their breasts—these are memories like no others.

At the time, though, these same mothers probably longed to get a full night's sleep. For infants, especially very young ones, waking up hungry several times a night is completely normal. Babies have small stomachs, and they're eating enough to triple their body weight within a year. This rapid rate of growth requires frequent feedings. A baby is not made to "sleep through the night." Dealing with this requires creativity, patience, and—sorry, Mom—acceptance.

Your baby craves not only your milk but the soothing closeness of your body. She was warm and cozy in your womb, and now she finds herself adrift in noisy, boundless life on the outside. She naturally stirs at night and seeks your breast for nutrition and comfort. She craves your familiar smell, touch, and presence. To deny your baby what she needs, biologically and psychologically, would be unnatural and counterproductive. The damage could be lasting, too, since avoiding night feedings or delegating them to your partner would send a mixed message to your body and disrupt your milk production.

Mothers who formula-feed often brag that their babies sleep through the entire night, but in our experience this isn't as common as people think. We see as many formula-feeding mothers as breastfeeding mothers struggle with sleep problems. In general, though, bottle-fed babies do sleep for longer stretches at a time than breast-fed babies. In fact, breastfed babies sleep less overall.

Marsha Walker, a lactation consultant and educator, points out that babies who are formula-fed from birth have "poor vagal tone." She is referring to the vagus nerve, which controls numerous sensations and reflexes throughout the body. In short, says Walker, formula-fed babies' autonomic nervous systems are measurably disordered. This makes them sleepier and less alert than breastfed newborns. (Poor vagal tone, by the way, is also related to inferior motor and mental development for at least two years after birth.)

In addition, when bottle-feeding is strictly scheduled, some babies respond by "shutting down." Eventually, they sleep for long stretches, even during growth spurts and other developmental stages when they would normally wake at night.

Your baby needs your milk and your presence, not necessarily in that order. Meeting your baby's nighttime needs is not a form of spoiling. Think how you would feel if you were alone in a new environment, hungry, wet, and just wanting to be held by the only source of comfort you know.

You will probably live for well more than half a million hours. Those few you spend rocking and nursing your babies in the night don't account for much of this time. You've already met the extreme demands of pregnancy and childbirth. Now understand that meeting your baby's nighttime needs is a normal and necessary part of motherhood.

To have the patience and energy to be available during the wee hours, it only makes sense to rest up during the day. People often advise new mothers to "nap when the baby naps," but few women heed this good advice. When your baby naps, you'll probably want to catch up on everything else you've been neglecting. Resist the urge. You are not an invalid, but you need to conserve your energy. Divvy up chores with your partner so you can take the naps you need.

Do what you can to make night feedings less taxing. Once you get the knack of nursing your baby while you're sitting down, learn to nurse lying down. This will make nighttime feedings much easier. People may tell you never to sleep with your baby, or warn you that you could roll over on your baby if you nurse lying down. It is prudent to nurse on a flat surface without bulky bedclothes and pillows around, but don't forego nursing while lying on your side. This is a natural position that women have instinctively adopted since the beginning of time. If you're worried you'll smother the baby, you can buy a Co-Sleeper, a baby bed that attaches to an adult bed so you can slide the baby back and forth without getting up. If you'd rather not nurse lying down, put a comfortable chair, changing supplies, and the baby's bed near your bed. Having all the essentials nearby will let you nurse and burp your baby and change a diaper, if needed, and be back to dreamland before you know it.

Suppose your baby doesn't go right back to sleep after nursing. Every baby is different. Among our own four nurslings, there were nurse-and-nappers, who went right back to sleep after they were fed, and night owls, who disregarded the sun. Some babies really do have their alert and interactive times at night, and in the early weeks there may be nothing you can do to change the situation. But you can shorten the active intervals by avoiding stimulating the baby. Don't sing or talk to her; don't rock her. Keep the lighting low, if not off completely. Use super-absorbent disposable diapers so she'll be able to wait for a change until the rooster crows.

Take care of your own sleep needs, but learn to roll with your nighttime nurser. Enjoy the quiet, priceless moments when the two of you are half-awake together in the darkness. Remember, this phase of life won't last long.

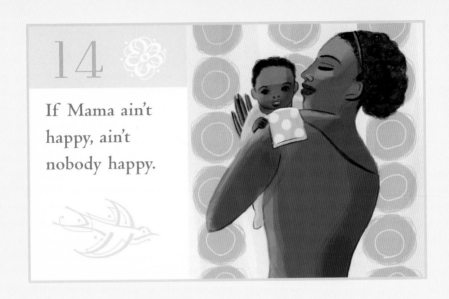

14

If Mama ain't happy, ain't nobody happy.

Have you ever watched the ripple effect from a rock thrown in the water? One big plunk sends waves in every direction. The far-reaching ones are subtle but still noticeable. An unhappy mother is like the rock that went plunk. Her mood and her state of mind spread out through the entire family. Simply put, if Mama ain't happy, ain't nobody happy.

Fatigue and anxiety can affect your immune system and your ability to recover after pregnancy and birth. And how can you heap love on your new baby if you're in physical or psychological discomfort?

After delivery, sleep deprivation usually conspires with physical and hormonal changes to cause a few days of the "baby blues." This common experience doesn't mean you're on a downward slide. But you do need to make a conscious effort to take care of yourself. This doesn't mean sitting around eating bonbons and having facials (though that sounds tempting, doesn't it?), but be aware that when you're preoccupied with baby care and trying to run your household you can easily end up neglecting yourself. And that would be bad for you and for your baby.

Protecting yourself from unhappiness isn't selfish. Think of the oxygen-mask rule: If you don't put your mask on first, you won't be able to help anyone else. Self-sacrifice is a common side effect of motherhood. Don't automatically put your needs last.

Struggles with breastfeeding are sometimes part of the hamster wheel of anxiety and exhaustion in early motherhood. This is one more reason you should get help as soon as possible if you have breastfeeding problems. During your early attempts at nursing, your friends may tell you, "Give it several weeks to get better." They're correct, but they don't mean you should go without professional guidance. Your sore nipples will not magically heal or your milk supply spring forth from the heavens. The tincture of time may not be enough if you are in pain or your baby is not growing.

We used to joke that a supermom is one who can shave both legs on the same day. You can forget about your hairy legs, but you really should get up and shower, comb your hair, and brush your teeth every day. Once you have a baby, you need to do these things after the first morning feeding, or it may be dinnertime before you know it!

As we have discussed already, rest and shut-eye are also important to a positive outlook. So are physical exercise and nutritious, high-protein meals. Omega-3 fatty acids have been shown to be valuable in decreasing postpartum depression.

Take a serious look at your food and fluid intake. Are you just grazing or eating a lot of "empty calories"? Are you scraping the leftovers off your older kid's plate and calling that dinner?

The traditional rule of thumb is that nursing mothers need 500 to 750 calories per day more than they needed before pregnancy. We believe that individual metabolic rates vary too greatly for this narrow range to apply to every nursing mother. Providing you established good eating habits and gained adequate weight during pregnancy, you probably won't need to change your diet much at all. You will need to drink more fluids, but just to quench your thirst and produce clear urine. Contrary to popular belief, drinking beyond the satisfaction of thirst does not increase milk production. You do not have to wear a cooler full of drinks around your neck.

New mothers commonly ask, "What can I eat?" There are no foods that nursing mothers should routinely avoid, although on occasion a baby will be bothered by something the mother has eaten (see Chapter 16). Unless your baby has unusual and persistent symptoms—

such as a sudden refusal to nurse, vomiting, diarrhea or green stools, gassiness or colic—chalk up any fussiness to "letting off steam." With moderation, you can indulge in coffee, tea, chocolate, cheeses, and sushi, and you can even enjoy an occasional glass of wine or beer. *That* should make Mama happy.

You may feel discouraged that your shape has not sprung back to normal after nine months of pregnancy. Give yourself a break. You lost some weight when you delivered, but you are probably months away from being back to your usual weight. Taking pounds off slowly, as nursing mothers tend to do naturally, is the best way to lose weight. Avoid crash diets; they can drain you of energy and stamina.

Contributing to the feeling that you are not quite yourself may be isolation, especially if you've left work or school—and most of your friends—to care for the baby. But your love for your baby doesn't lessen any craving you may have for adult companionship. If you have had a career outside the house, staying home much of the day will be a real change of pace. It may take some effort to relax and enjoy this respite from work.

Do get out, *with* your baby. Attend La Leche League meetings or infant massage classes, or, after the first month, enroll in a mother-baby exercise class. Socializing with women from your childbirth class is another excellent way to avoid isolation.

Having a clutter-free house could brighten your outlook, but at what price? Remember this old rhyme: "Trying to clean house while your children are growing is like trying to rake leaves while the wind is blowing!" As long as you can find the baby, your phone, and the television remote, and the house is only messy rather than really dirty, don't sweat the small household stuff. If someone offers to come and help you clean, though, don't hesitate to take them up on the offer.

As long as you're on your own, do housework a little at a time. Set reasonable goals—a few small cleanup tasks in one room per day. Figure out what makes you feel better nested and rested—a clear kitchen counter? a sparkling bathroom?—and work toward that end. Your mothering days will be over soon, but housework will always be there waiting. Take care of your own needs first, and you'll be better able to care for your family's.

Remember, keep Mama happy!

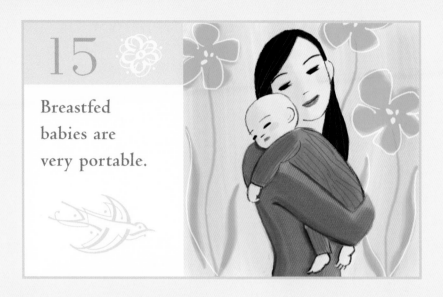

15

Breastfed babies are very portable.

I f you think breastfeeding is going to tie you down, you are very mistaken. Breastfeeding doesn't trap you in the house. In fact, once breastfeeding is going well, all you'll need to hit the road is your baby, your breasts, a couple of diapers, and a few moist wipes. Compare that to packing up bottles, formula, coolants, and warmers every time you leave the house, and you'll see the advantages. In many ways, nursing simplifies life considerably.

Of course, not everybody sees it this way. People may tell you that you should hire a babysitter so you will be able to get out without lugging the baby with you wherever you go. The inescapable truth is that your baby needs your presence as long as you're capable of providing it. By being near your nursling, you can provide for her most elemental needs, both physical and emotional.

Don't think of nursing as a barrier to mobility. Your luggage is light, and you are your baby's favorite traveling companion.

But maybe you feel uneasy about nursing your baby away from the comforts and privacy of your home. If you are going to be away for just a few hours, you may want to nurse just before you leave; this way, you may not need to nurse again until you're back home. If you're visiting friends or family, you can retreat to a bedroom to nurse, if that makes you comfortable. In public places, you could head to a ladies' room or changing room, but they aren't always handy or comfortable. And when you're along with friends and family you may not want to leave the party. So it's best to master a few simple tricks that will let you nurse inconspicuously and modestly.

At home, practice latching your baby onto your breast with a blanket or shawl draped over your shoulder and the baby's head. Nurse facing a mirror so you can see what others can (or can't) see. When you're out, you can use your baby sling or other wearable carrier like a cape both to maintain your privacy and to keep the baby from being distracted by activities around you. Soon you may find that you don't need a blanket or other covering if you wear a pullover shirt or sweater and pull it up from the bottom to nurse. Likewise, unbuttoning a blouse from the bottom rather than the top will expose less of your skin. Check the Internet for camisoles and tops specially designed for discreet nursing.

Keep in mind that you're not doing anything revolutionary. Every day, we're bombarded with images of cleavage on billboards, on TV, and in other media. You are using your breasts for their intended purpose. Learning to nurse discreetly and without embarrassment will put you, your partner, and most other people around you at ease.

Breastfeeding is also convenient on longer trips, whether you're driving or flying. Most young infants travel well in the car. The older baby may be less contented in the car seat for long periods. But you can buy yourself some peaceful traveling if you tank up the car *and* the baby before you leave.

If you're flying, try to reserve bulkhead seating, which will afford you more room and possibly more privacy. Nursing your baby during takeoff and landing will help her ears adjust to the changing air pressure in the cabin. This means less pain and less crying. Your fellow travelers will appreciate how fast you can meet her needs. If you experience travel delays, you can keep feeding your baby from a milk supply that never spoils or runs out, and keep her calm and secure, too.

Don't let your new baby clip your wings. Today's typical nursing mother is out and about, taking care of business, enjoying the company of friends, returning to work or school, and having fun. Take advantage of your nursling's portability. She will hit the ground running before you know it.

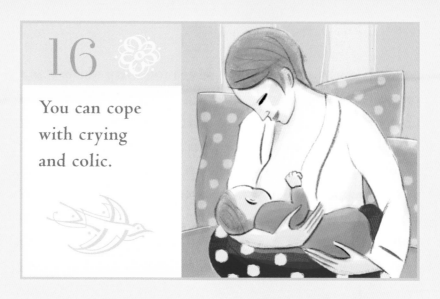

16

You can cope with crying and colic.

You may be amazed at how much your baby can cry. And you may be surprised how uncomfortable the crying makes you feel. When your baby cries, your mother-radar kicks in; you want to find out what's wrong and fix it. His cries are *supposed* to distress you; they're the only way he has to ask for help.

All babies fuss to some extent. Your baby may spend the first few days after birth just eating and sleeping, so when he perks up and

If you have an overabundant milk supply, an unusually fast flow, or both, your baby will tend to ingest mostly watery, lactose-rich foremilk. Too much foremilk causes tummy cramps, gas, and explosive stools. In this case, talk with your lactation specialist about possibly offering only one breast per feeding. This could reduce your production and ensure that your baby gets more hindmilk at each feeding.

While you are breastfeeding, your baby indirectly eats what you eat. It's possible that something in your diet may be bothering him. This doesn't mean that your baby might be allergic to your milk, but that he may be reacting to a protein in your diet. The usual suspects in such cases are dairy products, spices, gas-producing vegetables, and citrus. Caffeine and chocolate can cause problems for some babies, as well.

If your baby has blood or mucus in the stool, consult a doctor or lactation specialist. Otherwise, you might try to identify the problem yourself. Keep a food diary to help you correlate what you have eaten with bouts of crying. Then, if you suspect a particular food, omit it from your diet for at least three days. If your baby's discomfort goes away, you may have found the culprit. If he continues to cry, you might try omitting dairy products from your diet for two weeks, since milk proteins can take this long to clear from your system.

You should also consider anything else you or your baby ingests, directly or indirectly. If you're taking herbal supplements or any medications, including laxatives, you should consider them possible culprits. Sometimes a vitamin or fluoride supplement prescribed to a baby can cause fussiness as well.

One clue to a baby's distress that you can't possibly miss is gastric reflux, or spitting up. If your baby is fairly happy, spitting up is a laundry problem, not a baby problem. But if your baby is fussy after feedings, regularly spits up about thirty minutes afterward, resists lying flat on his back, has sour-milk breath, arches his neck and back, and acts hungry when you know he is well-fed, he may be experiencing severe reflux and heartburn. His doctor can diagnose this problem and may recommend treating it with medication.

If no one can identify a simple reason why a baby cries a lot, his troubles get lumped into the catch-all diagnosis colic, a condition that strikes fear in the hearts of new parents. It is characterized by periods of intense crying and apparent abdominal pain. Often crying spells occur in the late afternoon and evening, just as Mom's energy level ebbs and Dad hits the doorstep after a long day at work.

The causes of colic have been much debated over the years, but, alas for long-suffering parents, doctors have ultimately dismissed it as something parents simply have to endure until the baby is three to four months old. At around that age, the symptoms are expected to begin disappearing.

In the meantime, if your baby is unhappy, so are you. You're tired, disappointed, and upset. You can't plan a meal or even a shower without considering the needs of your complaining infant. Living with a colicky baby is stressful for everyone in the family, but the brunt of the misery usually falls on the mother, who constantly tries to soothe her child and identify the cause of his discomfort.

Parents of crying babies are deluged with tips for dealing with their infants. Tricks that are worth trying include exposing your baby to "white noise," putting him in a swing or a bouncy seat that vibrates, driving him around in the car, and administering "gas drops" (simethicone) or an infusion of ginger or fennel. "Wearing" your baby in a sling or front carrier is a good way to soothe him while still being able to move about and have your hands free. Both you and your baby will benefit from a change of scenery, so go outside and get some exercise.

It's difficult for relatives and friends to understand your problem if they haven't dealt with a colicky baby themselves. You may have to be adamant about your inability to be a hostess during this time. But you may also need to have people come in to help during your baby's predictably worst time of day. Others can take shifts walking and soothing your baby. If he prefers you or your partner, delegate chores and errands to volunteers.

Dealing with a colicky baby is probably not how you envisioned motherhood. Many mothers look back on their children's infancy as a big blur because of their babies' chronic crying and fussiness. Having had colicky babies ourselves, we know the fatigue and confusion colic visits on mothers. Keep seeking the causes of your baby's discomfort. You may not be able to cure him, but you can make him more comfortable.

And take good care of yourself. Get support from other mothers with whom you can talk openly about your stress. Grab every opportunity to rest. Make sure your partner takes turns soothing the baby.

Enjoy your baby's respites from crying. He is still lovable, even if he's challenging to care for. He will get better, in time. Until then, if you can cope, your baby can cope, too.

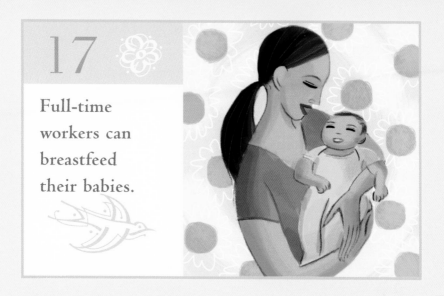

17

Full-time workers can breastfeed their babies.

Not so many years ago, if you were planning to return to work, you might never have considered nursing your baby beyond your maternity leave. Many women used to bottle-feed because they assumed breastfeeding would be impossible at work or school.

Even today, many working women have second thoughts about

breastfeeding. They fear being seen as unprofessional or as not pulling their weight on the job if they have to excuse themselves to pump their breasts two or three times a day. Some also worry that they'll have a harder time leaving the baby at home if they have established the close bond that comes with breastfeeding.

Yet, with the increased general awareness that breastfeeding is the best way to feed a baby, more and more mothers are opting to nurse their babies while continuing with their careers. Thanks to the legion of nursing mothers in the workplace, employers have taken notice. Recognizing that nursing mothers have generally healthier babies and so take less time off to care for sick children, they make nursing rooms or pump stations available. Some large companies even have lactation consultants on site. Others provide new mothers with a free pump along with access to lactation advice. The mothers appreciate these perks, which in turn makes them happier and more productive on the job. In a sense, breast milk is lubricating the wheels of industry.

Still, many workplaces lack designated rooms where a woman can pump her breasts in privacy. If this is the case with your company, ask your supervisor if there might be any private place where you can express your milk. We hope that, by the time you read this, there will be a federal law that protects a mother's right to express her milk or have her baby brought to her to nurse in the workplace. Until then, where there's a will there's a way.

Continuing to breastfeed while you work requires some careful planning, beginning well in advance of your first day back. Before you worry about the logistics of pumping and storing milk, decide when you want to go back to work and for how many hours. Breastfeeding experts have found that women who stay home for sixteen weeks or longer experience fewer difficulties maintaining their milk supplies. Can you extend your maternity leave? Can you work part time?

Some mothers who return to work part time prefer to continue part-time hours through their children's school years. Others start out working a few hours per week and gradually increase their hours until they are working full time again. Some jobs can be done from home, by telecommuting. Some women share jobs with other employees.

You must also decide who will take care of your baby. When you interview caregivers, tell each of them about your nursing relationship and your own particular style of caring for your baby. Make sure the caregiver respects your preferences; she should never take over as the expert on your baby. It may take a while to find someone who is compatible with your parenting values and who is affordable, available, and convenient to your home, workplace, or both. Follow your instincts; don't settle for anyone you have any reservations about.

If you will be missing one or more feedings while you are away at work or school, you should plan to express your milk (see Chapter 18 and Chapter 19). This will help prevent engorgement and, more important, maintain your milk supply. The milk you express can be used to feed your baby the next time you are separated. Once your baby is older than six months and taking solid foods, you may be able to go longer periods without pumping while continuing to nurse when you are together with your baby.

Breastfeeding offers you emotional compensation for the hours spent apart from your baby. A mother of twins remarked, "I looked forward all day to getting home and putting my feet up and nursing the girls!" You will feel the same way if you plan ahead and maintain your commitment to do the best for your baby.

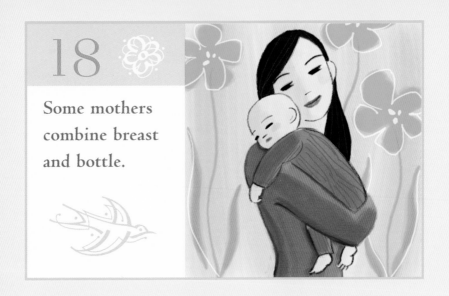

18

Some mothers combine breast and bottle.

Maybe you would like to start out breastfeeding but wonder how long you can continue. Some people may tell you that breastfeeding is easy and natural, but then you read about possible difficulties and complicated rules to follow. The prospect of committing yourself to six months of exclusive breastfeeding can be intimidating, especially if you're planning to return to work or school just a month or two after your baby's birth.

You may be relieved to know that, once you establish your milk supply, you can make adjustments to your feeding routines to suit your needs as well as your baby's. Many women combine breast- and bottle-feeding. Nursing is not an all-or-nothing endeavor.

If you're planning to return to work after a maternity leave, you'll want to establish a routine of breastfeedings interspersed with pumping sessions and bottle-feedings while you're home. This will make the transition easier for your baby when you return to work.

It's best to ease into a breast-bottle pattern. Nurse your baby exclusively for the first few weeks after his birth. While he is learning how to latch on to your breast, you don't want to confuse him with a bottle nipple.

When your milk is flowing well and your baby latches on to your breast automatically, you can begin occasionally offering him expressed breast milk from bottles. Begin by pumping milk after early-morning feedings, when you are likely to have a fuller milk supply. Offer this milk to your baby from a bottle later in the day to acclimate her to this delivery method. You can freeze excess pumped milk for later use, when you're getting the hang of pumping at work or when your baby is extra hungry.

There is an art to bottle-feeding a breastfed baby. Hold the baby in a sitting position and feed him in small amounts, stopping and starting in the relaxed way that he takes milk from your breast. If you instead allow your baby to guzzle milk from a bottle while lying flat on his back, he may come to expect this faster delivery and balk when milk from your breast doesn't flow as swiftly.

When you return to work, your baby may take so much milk from bottles that you have trouble pumping enough to keep up with his needs. If it's difficult for you to provide enough milk for all of your baby's daytime feedings, consider allowing the baby to have just enough formula to make up the difference. After the pressure to keep up with the baby's intake is lifted, some women relax and continue nursing for a long time. Remember, any amount of breast milk is better than none at all.

Some babies take relatively little milk when their mothers are away during the day but make up for the loss, nutritionally and emotionally, through frequent nursings during the evening and night. You might be surprised at how many women cope with this situation quite satisfactorily by keeping their babies close at hand all night and nursing while lying down.

Some mothers, employed or not, require uninterrupted nights' sleep to stay healthy and alert. Assuming your partner agrees to take on night feedings, you can get the sleep you need by pumping your breasts before you go to bed and then again, at your bedside, five or six hours later. Store the expressed milk in a bottle at room temperature for the next night feeding or until morning. The interruption will cost you only about fifteen minutes of sleep; you'll be back to sawing logs in no time.

Try not to go longer than six hours without draining your breasts, by nursing or pumping. This way, you'll not only avoid the discomfort of engorgement and reduce the risk of plugged milk ducts, which can lead to infections, but you'll ensure that your milk supply keeps up with your baby's appetite. Later on, when the baby takes longer breaks between feedings, you can pump less frequently.

Some women feed their babies breast milk exclusively from bottles, either because the baby simply doesn't learn to latch on to the breast or because, for one reason or another, the mother actually prefers this feeding method. Many women who do this have managed to produce enough milk to meet their babies' needs for months or even a year or longer.

Bottle-feeding breast milk full time requires dedication and discipline. It is a real labor of love. Unlike a baby, a pump doesn't cry for attention, and for most women, pumping is more a chore than a pleasure.

You can streamline the process by using an efficient electric breast pump that pumps both sides at once (see Chapter 19) and by adhering to a schedule that accommodates both your daily commitments and your baby's well-being. You'll need to pump more often during your child's natural growth spurts. At other times, you'll need to take care to avoid overfeeding, since babies often will take more milk from a bottle than they would from the breast. With this feeding plan, you will want the guidance of an expert counselor.

There are several approaches to combination feeding. Once you've gotten off to a good start with breastfeeding, you can choose the option that works best for you and your baby. Whether you feed him your milk directly, from a bottle, or both, and whether or not you supplement your milk with formula, you'll be giving your baby a vital gift.

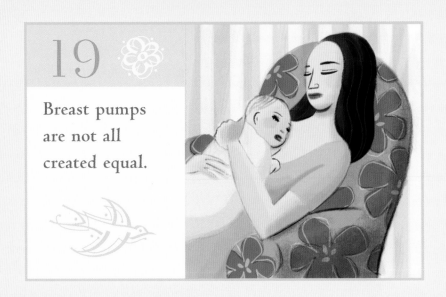

19

Breast pumps are not all created equal.

P umps have become a standard item on new mothers' "must have" lists. Many pregnant women buy the first model they find, and it ends up being inadequate. Others plunk down big bucks for a high-end model they'll never need. How do you know what kind of pump to buy, or whether to buy one at all?

There is a wide variety of pumps on the market, and their suitability depends on your particular needs. You may know your need only *after* your baby is born.

If you will be expressing your milk only occasionally, a small, portable manual pump, such as the Avent Isis, will suffice.

Many relatively inexpensive personal-use electric pumps are also available. These sell for less than $200 apiece, and most will run on either house current or batteries. A few of these pumps are designed to allow you to pump both breasts at the same time. Unfortunately, most bargain-priced electric pumps are a waste of money; they cycle too slowly to stimulate and drain the breasts effectively. An exception is Medela's single-sided Swing Pump, which runs on either house current or batteries. These pumps are great for a mom who will be apart from her baby for no more than a few feedings a week.

High-end personal-use pumps, such as Medela's Pump in Style series and Hollister's Purely Yours, have become very popular in recent years. But these models, designed for working moms, are more than many mothers need and less than others require. We recommend such pumps for mothers who have an adequate milk supply and will routinely miss a few nursings a day. Women who must pump only occasionally needn't invest in such heavy-duty equipment. Yet these models may be inadequate for women who, because of some complication, need to pump around the clock. These mothers should have a hospital-grade pump.

If you want a high-quality personal-use pump but don't want to pay the $250 to $350 price for it, you may be tempted to buy a used pump through eBay or borrow your sister-in-law's. We say, don't do it. Personal-use pumps are meant for one woman only; the U.S. Food and Drug Administration has labeled them more clearly as "single-user pumps." Although many women share, borrow, or sell these pumps, they can become contaminated and, at least in theory, can pass viruses from one mother to the next. In addition to hygienic concerns, a used pump may have lost some of its suction or speed.

If you buy a new pump, you'll get a one-year warranty. The full price may seem reasonable when you consider that it equals the cost of two to three months of infant formula. And you can use your pump with any other babies who come along, provided the suction and speed are still strong.

If you do not plan to take many outings away from your baby, you may not need a pump at all. Instead, you can learn how to express your milk manually. The technique is described in many books on breastfeeding and can be demonstrated by a lactation specialist. It takes a little practice, but hand expression can be very effective. Once you learn to do it, your "pump" is at the end of your arm.

If you're unsure whether to buy a pump or what kind to buy, you can rent one by the day, week, or month. Rental units are strong, reliable hospital-grade pumps, and each mother gets her own sterile collection kit.

If your baby is hospitalized, your insurance company may cover the cost of renting a hospital-grade pump (although you may have to fill out and file the paperwork yourself). If your baby can't nurse and your insurance company won't pay for pump rental, you may be able to use funds from a flex-spending account or medical savings account.

Breast pumps aren't suitable shower gifts, and they shouldn't be emergency purchases. A pump can have a profound impact on your nursing experience. Before deciding to purchase one, know your needs, and do some research. A lactation specialist can help evaluate your needs and make your choices clearer.

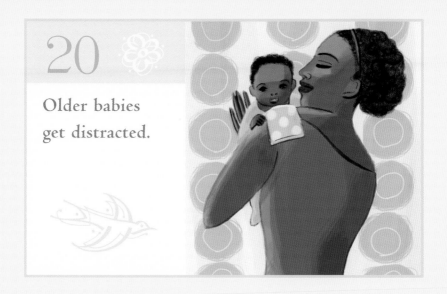

20

Older babies get distracted.

After your first few months with your baby, you will have settled into a fairly predictable routine. You'll be better acquainted with each other, and your baby may even have a somewhat regular nursing and sleeping routine. The early challenges of breastfeeding are in the past, and you are both eager to continue.

Not so fast! Just when you thought you were over the hump, your baby will enter a new challenging developmental stage. Anticipating this stage will help you adjust your breastfeeding relationship as needed without undue stress.

At about three to five months, your baby will become enamored with the world around her. While nursing, she will be easily distracted. She'll pull away from the breast at any new, sudden, or interesting sight or sound, look around, and try to find the source.

Older siblings and their friends can be a prime distraction at this stage. Your baby will be instantly excited by the uproar as they roughhouse and careen merrily through the house.

At around this age, too, your baby may start to play nursing games. She may stop sucking, for instance, to pat your face and smile. Although these antics are endearing, you may become frustrated if nursing sessions become longer because your baby never wants to get down to the business of breastfeeding.

And just when you have mastered the art of nursing in public, your baby turns into a lapful of squirming arms and legs. When you're sitting on a bench at the mall, you may not feel comfortable offering your breast to a moving target.

Your baby's distracted behavior doesn't mean she has lost interest in nursing. After several weeks of interrupted feedings, she will no longer have to let go of the nipple to check out what's going on around her. Instead, she'll turn her head with the nipple still in her mouth.

Especially if you are back in the workplace, you may be concerned that distracted, haphazard nursing will reduce your milk production. Your breasts will usually be softer now, and they will be less likely to feel engorged if you miss a feeding or if your baby sleeps longer than usual. Your milk may not let down as fast as it did in the early days. Your milk supply is naturally leveling off at this time because your baby's growth is slowing down, and it may slow even more if your baby is sporadically latching on and off. Irregular milk removal can indeed put your milk supply at risk.

If you're worried about this, or just frustrated by your baby's distractibility, try what some experienced mothers call "sheltered nursing." Take your baby into a quiet, dark room, preferably when she is sleepy. Rock or sway or even pace as you nurse. At night, try lying on your side to nurse in a darkened room. This way your baby will be less likely to pull the on-again, off-again routine that makes feedings longer and less productive.

To make up for decreased milk intake during the day, your baby may begin lengthening nighttime feedings—a trend you'll surely take as an ominous sign. Take heart. She will probably return to her regular schedule (which, of course, is always subject to change) when she passes through this distracted phase.

If sheltered nursing and longer night feedings don't boost your milk supply, you might try "insurance pumping"—a few extra pumping sessions to safeguard your milk production.

Patience may be all you need to cope with your baby's distracted behavior. If your milk supply is affected, though, do take care to protect it.

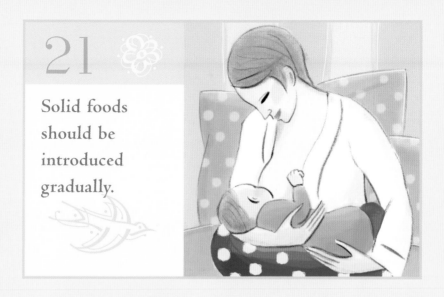

21

Solid foods should be introduced gradually.

During your baby's first year, every stage in his development is entertaining. This is especially true when he starts eating from a spoon instead of just from your breasts. You will enjoy watching him experiment with this new activity, even though it's often messy!

But don't rush to introduce solids before your baby is ready. He must be able to actually swallow and digest these foods.

At what age will he be able to do this? The American Academy of Pediatrics (AAP) advises introducing iron-rich foods gradually, beginning around six months of age, while continuing to breastfeed at least through the baby's first year. Some babies, the AAP says, may show a need for complementary foods as early as four months of age, but others may not be ready to accept other foods until about eight months.

As your baby approaches the middle of his first year, look for signs that he is ready for table foods. A baby shows readiness for solids by sitting up, reaching for food at the table, and otherwise acting interested in eating what his family eats.

Another sign of readiness is his appetite. When your baby is close to six months old, you may begin to notice that he still seems hungry after nursing. If after a few days of stepped-up nursings he still seems unsatisfied, feel free to experiment with solids. Occasionally a four- or five-month-old fails to gain sufficient weight, or stops gaining at all. Most babies between four and six months of age gain two to three ounces a week. If normal weight gain doesn't resume after a week or so of extra nursings, it may be time to begin solids.

Nurse your baby before offering cereal or another solid food. It is important to do this until she is eating three regular meals of table food, which usually happens sometime after eight months. Until then, breast milk should continue to be her main source of calories and nutrients.

So, how do you begin introducing solids? A variety of foods have been recommended as first solids, but an iron-fortified baby cereal mixed with breast milk meets both a baby's nutritional and his developmental needs. Cereal also meets the baby's increased need for iron that occurs at around six months.

Begin with one feeding of cereal a day. At first, mix one tablespoon of cereal with enough breast milk to make a thin paste. Initially, don't be surprised if your baby pushes back out almost as much as you have put in. Even though he may lunge for your plate, he may not have lost his extrusion reflex, which will cause him to thrust his tongue out rather than swallow. It may take a while before he learns to move the food to the back of his mouth for swallowing. Patience and practice will prevail if he is truly ready for solid food.

A variety of prepared, jarred foods are available for babies, but you may prefer mashing and mixing fresh vegetables and fruit yourself. Making your baby's food can be simple and economical. Avocados, sweet potatoes, and bananas are wonderful early foods that your baby can enjoy along with the entire family.

Resist the urge to spoon large amounts of jarred foods to your baby. For one thing, he needs to learn to pace his own meals and enjoy the social aspect of eating and playing with his food. Besides, if he fills up on solids your milk supply may be at risk at a time when he is developing gross motor skills (crawling, pulling up, and first steps) that can compete for breast time. Don't misinterpret his enthusiasm for these new adventures as a lack of interest in nursing.

When adding new foods to the baby's menu, offer one at a time so you can identify the source of any allergic reactions.

For more advice on feeding babies and toddlers, we recommend Ellyn Satter's *Child of Mine: Feeding with Love and Good Sense.*

Letting your baby take the lead from his cradle to the family table is the most logical and rewarding way to start your baby on solids. He will show you when he is ready. Then grab a bib, some wipes, a floor mat (or the family dog), and get started. Go slowly, and enjoy the process as he learns this new skill.

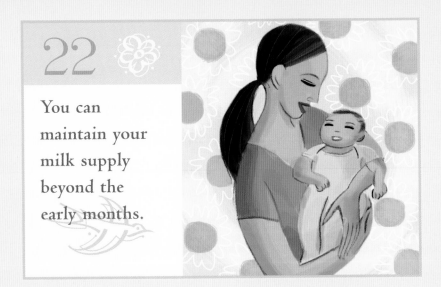

22

You can maintain your milk supply beyond the early months.

I n our practices, we often see the same mothers we counseled after childbirth come back several months later complaining that their baby has slowed down her nursing or that their milk supply seems to be drying up. Supply slumps are a common problem, but they can be overcome—and in many cases avoided.

Usually, the slowdown is normal. After four to five months, research has found, babies usually begin to gain weight more slowly. (Think about it: In the early days, a baby gains an ounce a day. If she kept this up, she'd hit thirty pounds by her first birthday!) Consequently, older babies' demand for milk doesn't increase as dramatically as it did before.

Some researchers think that breast milk meets a baby's changing needs with quality rather than quantity, by becoming richer in fat. Another theory holds that as a baby's digestive tract matures she becomes better able to absorb nutrients from the milk. Whatever the reason, a mother's milk supply apparently reaches a ceiling of twenty-four to thirty-two ounces per day. Yet, despite a baby's increased weight and advancing age, *she usually continues to grow.*

Sometimes, though, a mother's production declines. How can you tell if this is your problem? Mostly by watching your baby. She'll notice before you will, and she'll let you know by telling you how unsatisfied she is after nursings. If she squirms and pulls off the breast or wakes to nurse more often, your milk supply may have decreased. There can be other reasons for this behavior, but if you really feel your milk supply is low, you may want to take steps to increase it. (If you suspect your baby has stopped growing or is actually losing weight, consult a doctor or lactation specialist.)

The way to prompt your body to produce more milk is to raise the demand for it. For any of the reasons outlined below, your baby may not be asking for enough. Lessened nursing lowers production, and lower production may discourage her from nursing well. This is a vicious cycle that you want to avoid.

Distracted baby. As discussed in Chapter 20, your supply may dwindle because your baby is continually distracted from nursing. Try to minimize the ambient household chaos when you nurse.

Active baby. At six months, your baby's attentiveness to her hunger may suffer because she is preoccupied with crawling and otherwise mastering her floor-level domain. She may actually forget to ask for food. Offer her your breast when she isn't on a roll.

Striking baby. There's another first-year phenomenon that can take its toll on your milk supply: a nursing strike. Yes, your baby may suddenly simply boycott your breast. And it won't be because he's ready to be weaned (see Chapter 23). Rarely, babies wean themselves between eight and twelve months, but they usually do so gradually. A nursing strike is sudden.

Strikes usually occur after the first six months, but they can come at any time and for many reasons—teething, a cold, an ear infection, or a painful herpes infection in the mouth. They also sometimes surface following a prolonged separation of mother and baby or after a baby has bitten her mother and was frightened by Mom's cry of pain.

Sometimes we see strikes when a baby has become accustomed to a bottle and its immediate gratification. Her refusal to nurse is coupled with a decline in her mother's milk supply.

Nursing strikes typically last a few days, but they may go on for a few weeks. Most striking babies can be coaxed back to the breast. Rule out any infections or physical problems, and then use the same techniques recommended for winning back the attention of a distractible baby (see page 118). A strike can be upsetting, but don't take it personally. Your baby is not rejecting you; for some reason she is just shy about nursing. Through it all, protect your milk supply by pumping when you miss a nursing.

Frequent separations. If you work outside the home or go off to school for long periods, of course, you need to pump your breasts when you're away. If your supply drops, take advantage of every convenient opportunity to pump at school or work. When you're back with your baby, offer him your breast without restriction.

Sleeping baby. If your baby is sleeping for ten to twelve hours at night (don't mention this around brand-new mothers!) and taking a few catnaps and a longer nap during the day, you may find that your baby's nursing times and meal times all fall within about eight waking hours. As long as your baby is thriving you can let her sleep, but you may need to pump at your bedside to keep up your milk supply, especially if she is nursing less than five times a day.

Mom's meds. Sometimes medications can derail a milk supply. Birth-control pills that contain estrogen usually lower milk production. Progesterone-only oral contraceptives are less likely to affect supply, but some women have problems with these as well. Another group of drugs to avoid when possible are decongestants and antihistamines, which can have a drying effect on your milk supply.

Mom's cycle. When your menstrual cycle returns, you may notice a temporary change in your milk supply—probably a drop right before and during the first few days of menstruation. If your baby nurses poorly at this time, someone may tell you it's because your milk "tastes funny." More likely, she is reacting to the reduced milk supply.

When your baby, for whatever reason, stops nursing as often or as long or as vigorously, your first tactic should be to tempt her to nurse more. Take shirtless naps with her, wear her in a sling while you go about your business, or bring her into your bath. Avoid pacifier use; you want to be sure your baby isn't substituting non-nutritive sucking for nursing.

If your baby's nursing doesn't improve, you should, as we've said so often, express your milk to simulate higher demand.

Many mothers report an increase in milk supply when they pay better attention to their food and fluid intake. Prepare simple, nutritious foods early in the day when you have more energy, and avoid grabbing empty-calorie foods on the run. There is no need to drink when you're not thirsty, but keep water on hand so you'll have it when you need it.

If the tips here don't restore your milk supply, you can try herbal or prescription agents that stimulate milk production. The herb fenugreek works well. So do the prescription drugs Reglan and domperidone. We have seen dramatic turnarounds in women who combined these medications with extra feedings or pumpings. Talk with a lactation specialist or other health professional about these options if stepped-up feedings and pumpings don't help.

Your milk supply *can* be resurrected from a slump. Paying careful attention to your baby's signals and taking corrective measures promptly will ensure plenty of milk for your growing baby.

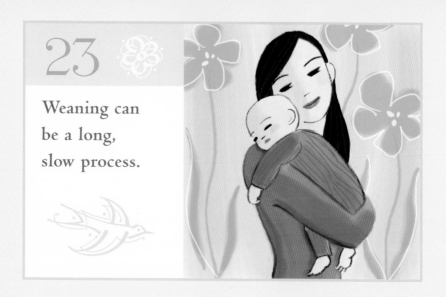

23

Weaning can
be a long,
slow process.

After every beginning comes an ending. The timing and technique may differ, but weaning from the breast is a major mothering milestone shared by all nursing mothers. It's often an emotional experience for women, laden with sadness as well as relief.

Weaning is usually a long, slow process. It begins when you first offer your baby solid food, but at this point, about halfway through your baby's first year, the end may still be far off. The American Academy of Pediatrics recommends nursing until a baby is *at least* one year old. La Leche League is less precise, suggesting only that you nurse until your baby "outgrows the need."

To a new or expectant mother, a year sounds like a long time to nurse. If you have never breastfed, it may be difficult to imagine nursing a baby who has teeth, who can walk, and who actually asks to be nursed. But consider that, unlike babes in arms, older babies don't nurse "all the time." You don't have to be an open buffet every minute of the day for an older nurser. Biting is occasionally a problem, but usually a short-lived one, when it occurs. Keep an open mind. You may be surprised at how long you nurse your little one.

Worldwide, the average weaning age is between two and four years. In North America, weaning is usually earlier. Women wean in the first year for a variety of reasons. There may be ongoing breastfeeding difficulties, a medical condition, a jealous partner or sibling, or another emotional problem involved. Some mothers wean when they get pregnant, return to work or school, go on a diet, plan a vacation, or simply feel it's time to move on. Those who are pumping and bottle-feeding all their milk may get tired of the routine. Other women tire of all the physical contact with their babies or of feeling "like a cow." Those whose babies deny them too much sleep just get tired, period.

In all of these cases, it's best if Mom can find a compromise that gives her a break but still provides her baby with some breast milk.

If you thought that breastfeeding was going to be entirely instinctive and easy, but have ended up with latch-on problems, sore nipples, low milk supply, or other breastfeeding difficulties, you may want to stop nursing after the first few weeks. At this early stage, you should seek out people who can help you before you simply stop breastfeeding.

Many women who call our help lines ask how to wean their

babies. Sometimes this is a subtle cry for help with breastfeeding problems. Other times, a mother has made up her mind to quit or is facing circumstances beyond her control. Whatever your reasons, if you ask for help with weaning your counselor shouldn't try to talk you into continuing breastfeeding your baby. It is *your* decision when to wean and why, and the people you ask for advice should respect that. You are not a bad mother for wanting to wean.

You should, however, expect the person on the other end of the line to ask specific questions to rule out problems that may not require total weaning and to suggest possible compromises. Partial formula-feeding may be the best solution. If you've decided that it's really time to stop nursing your child, the counselor should give you advice to make the process easier—emotionally and physically—on both you and baby.

It's worth making the call. Once you've considered all your options, you may end up feeling regret about early weaning, but at least you shouldn't feel guilty.

Weaning is best done gradually, by eliminating one daily feeding at a time. If your baby is younger than a year, you will need to replace your milk with formula; a baby older than a year can drink whole cow's milk. Gradual weaning allows you to maintain a backup milk supply while you make sure your baby has no negative reaction to formula or cow's milk. Introducing a bottle or cup while you're still breastfeeding also gives your baby time to learn the new feeding method without going hungry.

Your physical comfort is also a major consideration in weaning. The time it takes to "dry up" varies from mother to mother, but if you stop removing milk abruptly your breasts will likely become engorged, and you will risk plugged milk ducts and breast infection (mastitis). If instead you eliminate feedings gradually, your milk-producing cells will soon get the message that there's less demand for your milk, and your production will slowly decrease. "Don't offer, don't refuse," recommends La Leche League. This way you'll avoid ending your breastfeeding relationship abruptly, but you won't be encouraging it to drag on, either.

If for some reason you must wean your baby suddenly, there are ways to minimize your discomfort. Apply cold compresses or chilled green cabbage leaves to your breasts, wear a supportive bra that doesn't bind, and avoid warm showers and other stimulation. Some women take ibuprofen or some other pain reliever. Certain herbs, such as sage, peppermint, and parsley, are reputed to decrease milk production. If you are planning to begin taking an oral contraceptive, ask your doctor about a "combo pill" of estrogen and progesterone; it could help you reduce milk production. Talk to your doctor, though, before taking any drugs to promote weaning.

However and whenever you wean, you can make your baby more comfortable by providing other kinds of mothering—extra cuddles and attention to reassure him that you're still his source of comfort and solace.

Much additional advice on weaning is provided in *The Nursing Mother's Guide to Weaning: How to Bring Breastfeeding to a Gentle Close, and How to Decide When the Time Is Right* by Kathleen Huggins and Linda Ziedrich. The book stresses the standard weaning tactics of shortened nursings, postponement, substitution, and distraction. It also discusses an overlooked element of weaning: the safe preparation of formula.

As your nursing days come to a close, congratulate yourself on having provided your baby with the haven of your breast and your milk. Whether you have weaned against your will or gladly, recognize how great a gift you have given your baby.

In a sense, motherhood is a series of weanings. As with all child-rearing milestones, trust your intuition, consider everyone's needs, and seek expert guidance before making radical decisions. Your memories will be sweeter when you feel you have played an active role in making them.

24

You can mentor
other mothers.

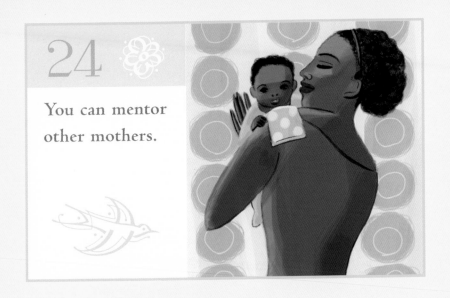

Not too many generations ago, nearly every new mother could turn to her own mother for guidance about breastfeeding. Fewer women can do this today. For many, the art of breastfeeding is learned alone—by trial and error, which all too often leads to frustration and discouragement.

Thankfully, during the past several decades mother-to-mother support groups have proliferated. Peer-counseling programs—most notably, La Leche League—have blossomed. Lactation consulting has been established as a profession, with a certifying board. The WIC (Special Supplemental Nutrition Program for Women, Infants, and Children) program now actively supports and promotes breast-feeding, and most communities have some sort of local breastfeeding support group.

You can play an important part in mother-to-mother support and information sharing. Once you master the skills and surmount the challenges of nursing, you'll be well suited to mentor other mothers who want to do the same. Every mother and every baby is different, but being a good listener and acknowledging that new motherhood is a time of adjustment and, on some days, disillusionment can mean the world to a struggling mom. You can reassure a mother that her ambivalent feelings are normal and not a sign that she doesn't love her baby enough—and she'll believe you.

Tell new moms funny stories about your own early days of motherhood. A good laugh can relieve the tension and anxiety that new mothers feel. When a mother of two-year-old twins told a group of new mothers of multiples that the perfect nursing chair had a padded toilet seat, water fountain, microwave, and TV attached, their nervousness melted way.

If a new mom shows feelings of despair, worthlessness, or anxiety, or if she can't sleep or has no appetite, you can play a vital role by urging her to seek professional help. You might help her make an appointment with a doctor or therapist who can rule out postpartum depression, and you might even drive her to the office. A woman in the midst of postpartum depression can't identify her feelings and usually won't ask for help. Intervene; she will thank you later.

You can also teach your baby's doctor about breastfeeding. If the doctor gives you breastfeeding advice, report back on whether it worked. If it did, let your doctor know how much you appreciate the help. If the doctor referred you to a lactation specialist, tell the doctor whether this made a difference for you and the baby. Good doctors constantly reassess their practices according to what they learn from patients. Sharing your experience will help ensure that, in the future, other mothers will get helpful advice.

Tell other mothers about the rewards of nursing. Describe listening to your baby's soft breathing at your breast as she drifts off to sleep. Tell about times when breastfeeding was convenient or even invaluable—during electrical outages, storms, and travel delays, for example. And note the pricelessness of the ability to comfort a sick child at your breast. Don't keep these things secret.

Give a thumbs-up to a mother you see quietly nursing in public. Or nod approval when she scans the room for detractors. Another mother is an oasis in a less-than-baby-friendly environment.

When you see a mother struggling to juggle her shopping cart, a wailing baby, and a diaper bag, look around and notice how many folks just step around the chaos. Then offer to help, or at least acknowledge her plight with a sympathetic smile.

If you have had difficulties nursing, yours will be a good shoulder to cry on for a mother who is undergoing similar struggles. You can understand her disappointment, anger, and grief. Just listening to her story will be a gift to her.

You are going to be part of the worldwide sorority of nursing mothers. Membership comes with privileges and responsibility. Your prebaby notions of motherhood and breastfeeding will have changed, and you will have knowledge to share. We may lack the multigenerational family life that mothers enjoyed in decades gone by, but we can still support and guide one another. So take your place in the breastfeeding sisterhood by lighting the next candle of hope, inspiration, and understanding. Mentor on.

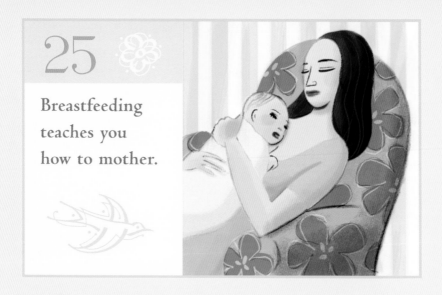

25

Breastfeeding teaches you how to mother.

The slogan of the U.S. National Breastfeeding Awareness Campaign is "Babies were born to be breastfed." But not all babies are fortunate enough to experience that birthright. To those of us in the business of supporting breastfeeding, nursing is more than just the source of milk of unparalleled value. It's a way of mothering your baby. In many respects, breastfeeding teaches you how to mother.

You may learn how to diaper, burp, and swaddle a baby before you give birth, but only afterward will you really learn to meet her physical and emotional needs. You will know when and how to respond to your baby because of your unique connection to her. And that precious relationship begins at the breast.

When breastfeeding begins, your baby will learn the sound of your voice, the taste of your milk, the smell of your skin, and the comfort of your embrace. You quickly become sensitive to her cues and signals. Your loving breastfeeding partnership is your tutorial for motherhood. Nursing mothers become experts on their babies.

At first you'll be unsure of your ability to decipher your baby's demands and responses, but before long you and the baby will share your own special ways of communicating. Often unconsciously, you will adjust your mothering style to meet needs your baby can't verbalize. You will learn her likes and dislikes. Each day you both grow and discover more.

As you respond to your baby by giving her what she needs, your baby learns to trust. She begins to smile and coo, rewarding you for your efforts. Before long, you'll be playing games and singing together.

Your intimacy with your baby will help you meet the many demands of motherhood. You will learn patience and gentleness. You will gain confidence. You will learn to put the baby's needs before your own. You'll learn that you are stronger than you think. Above all, you will build a relationship of trust and communication that will last a lifetime.

Exactly how you make this journey will be an experience as individual as your baby. Breastfeeding gives you the foundation to find what fits. Some families practice "attachment parenting," defined by Bill and Martha Sears (a pediatrician and a nurse and coauthors of several books on baby care) as a parenting style that "includes closeness right from birth, responding sensitively to cries, baby-wearing, sharing sleep, and breastfeeding." Other families find their own ways of accommodating the baby's needs and allowing Mom to breastfeed as much and as long as possible.

There is no single right way to mother your baby; if your baby is loved and protected, you're doing fine. However you care for your child, the breast milk you provide and the time you spend breastfeeding will be a great gift for both of you.

You are your baby's rock in a sea of change. You have earned her trust while nourishing her at your breast. All she knows of human relationships originates with you. Being able to protect and comfort your baby is one of the best feelings in the world. It is our legacy as women and our biological destiny.

No scientific breakthrough can replace the loving arms of a mother or the perfect milk from her breasts. Breastfeeding is truly a gift of love and connection. Savor your baby's early years. You will cherish the memories for a lifetime.

Recommended Reading

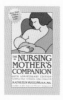*The Nursing Mother's Companion*, 20th Anniversary Edition, by Kathleen Huggins, The Harvard Common Press, 2005. Kathleen Huggins's complete, up-to-date guide to nursing, with easy-reference Survival Guide chapter for problem solving and an appendix on the safety of using various drugs during breast-feeding. See www.nursingmotherscompanion.com for more information.

OTHER NOTEWORTHY BOOKS

Gromada, Karen Kerkhoff. *Mothering Multiples: Breastfeeding & Caring for Twins or More*, 3rd rev. ed. Schaumburg, Ill.: La Leche League International, 2007.

Huggins, Kathleen, and Linda Ziedrich. *The Nursing Mother's Guide to Weaning: How to Bring Breastfeeding to a Gentle Close, and How to Decide When the Time Is Right*, rev. ed. Boston: Harvard Common Press, 2007.

Karp, Harvey. *The Happiest Baby on the Block: The New Way to Calm Crying and Help Your Newborn Baby Sleep Longer.* New York: Bantam Books, 2003.

La Leche League International. *The Womanly Art of Breastfeeding,* 7th rev. ed. Schaumburg, Ill.: La Leche League International, 2004.

Satter, Ellyn. *Child of Mine: Feeding with Love and Good Sense,* 3rd rev. ed. Boulder: Bull Publishing, 2000.

Sears, Martha, and William Sears. *25 Things Every New Mother Should Know.* Boston: Harvard Common Press, 2005.

Sears, Robert W., and James M. Sears. *Father's First Steps: 25 Things Every New Dad Should Know.* Boston: Harvard Common Press, 2006.

Sears, William, and Martha Sears. *The Attachment Parenting Book: A Commonsense Guide to Understanding and Nurturing Your Baby.* Boston: Little, Brown, 2001.

West, Diana, and Lisa Marasco. *The Breastfeeding Mother's Guide to Making More Milk.* New York: McGraw-Hill, 2008.

About the Authors

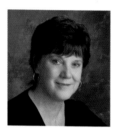 Kathleen Huggins, R.N., M.S., I.B.C.L.C., is a registered nurse and board-certified lactation consultant who has dedicated her career to helping mothers care more effectively for their newborn babies. She is the author of the best-selling classic book on breastfeeding *The Nursing Mother's Companion*. She is also the author of *The Expectant Parents' Companion* and is coauthor of *The Nursing Mother's Guide to Weaning* and *Nursing Mother, Working Mother*. She lives in San Luis Obispo, California, with her husband and youngest child.

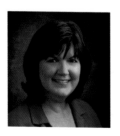 Jan Ellen Brown, I.B.C.L.C., is a board-certified lactation consultant who, over the past 20 years, has helped countless families meet their breastfeeding goals. A retired La Leche League leader and mother of two daughters, she gives frequent lectures on breastfeeding and parenting issues and practices with a pediatric group. She lives and works in Charlotte, North Carolina.